Pain case studies
With
Distal acupuncture

A week in a
Tung acupuncture
clinic

Published by: Draycott Publishing

Copyright © 2015 by Deborah Bleecker and Brad Whisnant
1st Edition

The author of this book does not dispense medical advice or prescribe the use of any technique as a form of treatment for physical, emotional, or medical problems without the advice of a physician, either directly or indirectly. The intent of the authors is only to offer information of a general nature to help you in your quest for emotional and spiritual well-being. In the event you use any of the information in this book for yourself, which is your constitutional right, the author and the publisher assume no responsibility for your actions.

The names and other identifying characteristics of the people in this book have been changed.

ISBN-978-1-940146-09-6

Pain
Case studies
With
Distal acupuncture

A week in a tung
Acupuncture clinic

Brad Whisnant, L.Ac., D.A.O.M.
Deborah Bleecker, L.Ac., M.S.O.M.

Acknowledgements

This book is only possible because of all the people who helped me and spent time with me.

I am grateful to Dr. Tan. I took many of his classes, and followed him in his clinic. He has been very generous with his time. Without him, "distal" acupuncture would not be as well known. Because of his tireless efforts over thirty years, we are able to learn this type of acupuncture, for which we are all thankful.

Dr. Wei Chieh Young has been so generous in his teachings. I can honestly say that although I have put this book together, without either of these two masters, I would not have been able to write this book.

It is because of these two individuals that so many of us have success in our clinics and are able to help others. I am grateful that I was lucky enough to spend time with these doctors.

Thank you.

There is only one way to avoid criticism: do nothing, say nothing, and be nothing.

–Aristotle

CONTENTS

A life spent making mistakes is not only more honorable, but more useful than a life spent doing nothing.

George Bernard Shaw

INTRODUCTION

The case studies in this book are about pain. A few of the cases are about pain that has another root, such as face pain from inflamed sinuses, or back pain from an inflamed liver. I have tried to show different types of pain. All of these case studies were taken from a seven-day period at my clinic. Some of these patients were new, and some were old. Some were easy, and some were difficult. Some patients were on board with treatment, and some were coming just because someone told them to.

Some of these patients had health insurance coverage, so paying for their care was not a concern. Some are very poor, and do not have many healthcare options. Some were coming back for maintenance, and others had a recovery with one treatment. This is much like any of your clinics.

This is how it is in a real acupuncture clinic. This is how it is every day in my clinic. I treat all my patients myself. I do not hire interns, and I do not treat community style. I have three treatment rooms. I spend about an hour and a half on new patients. A return visit is 45 minutes. Sometimes, if I am too busy and there are no treatment rooms available, I will treat people in the waiting area for a few minutes.

I think we can all agree the most common types of pain we see in acupuncture clinics are: Back, neck, shoulder, knee, headaches, fingers and toes, trauma, sciatica, low back pain, and the pains that no one else can fix. Of course there are many different types of pain as there are people, but usually, again the 80-20 rule (80% of the time you will be treating the same 20% of diseases).

As you read these cases, please note that the pain is not always the core issue. In some cases, there is another cause.

My first experience of this was my godfather. He painted a fence on Friday. Monday morning he had back pain. I was around 20 at the time, before I studied Chinese medicine. He went to his medical doctor for a routine evaluation for his back pain, and discovered it was actually stage four pancreatic cancer. He died two weeks later.

Pain is sometimes just that, pain. It's just inflammation, Qi and blood stagnation, dampness, heat, vaso-constriction, degeneration, your basic normal pain stuff.

In some cases, pain can be a warning that something serious is going on. If pain does not go away or change after acupuncture, it always bothers me. Acupuncture is so good, and so amazing, that if the patient does not feel any change in three to four visits, you can almost use that as a diagnostic tool.

In most cases, if you have treated someone three or four times, with no benefit, there are two possible reasons why. Either you did not do a correct diagnosis, or you used the wrong points. Another option is that the pain is a result of a serious disease.

I cannot tell you of all the times a pain did not go away, and it was a misdiagnosed broken bone, cancer, a scary virus, or something extremely dangerous. That doesn't mean I heal everyone. There are only two types who heal everyone, the devil and liars. I just wanted to emphasize that if you treat someone for pain and you get no change at all, there is a serious problem. You will need to investigate further.

It is extremely important to remember this when diagnosing back pain. Is it really back pain, or is it a problem with the bones, joints, muscles, tendons, or the discs? I could also be an inflamed liver, kidney stones, pain from menstruation, appendicitis, pancreatitis, splenitis, cancer, a blood clot, and an impacted bowel. There are many reasons why something can cause pain that is referred to the back.

Another example of this is a patient I treated recently. Her first treatment was for sacral pain. Her pain was 100% relieved while in my office. Three days later she called me back and said her pain had moved down into her groin. It felt like the pain would come and go and "roll through her."

It was my fault for not correctly checking the pulse, and asking enough questions. Upon further questioning, this patient had a history of kidney stones. She said she "felt just like the last time I had a stone." I referred her out for a CT scan and the diagnosis was confirmed, a kidney stone. This is a classic example of when back pain is not just back pain.

Although the back is just bones, muscles, and joints, it can be very difficult to treat. It is of utmost importance that we can treat back pain effectively. Over 85% of all acupuncture visits are for pain, in particular back pain.

Pain is so important to treat because 95% of the time patients will only come to us to treat pain. After patient education, and the patient feeling more comfortable with us, we have the chance to help them with other health issues. In their minds, if we cannot resolve the pain effectively, we certainly could not help them with other health problems.

Why These Case Studies

These case studies were chosen because I used only acupuncture on them. Most patients get acupuncture, herbs, cold laser, diet advice, etc. I used only Master Tung acupuncture in these cases. I wanted to show how using Tung acupuncture alone is sufficient. However, you will do better if you use Chinese herbs, give dietary advice, and add in some type of local stimulation. I use a cold laser. However, all of these cases were treated with just needles.

I do not heal every patient. I have treated patients for seven years, and given 65,000 treatments in multiple countries, using Tung acupuncture. I fail, learn, and continue to try. If I can be successful in my small town of 12,000 people, doing Tung acupuncture on all my patients, so can you. I am not special, I have no secrets, or golden needles. I have learned from studying, trying new things, observing, and learning from my failures. Anyone can do this with a little time and effort. I am a beginner.

This works in my small town, where no one likes, believes in, or wants to get acupuncture. I change my points regularly. I can have ten patients with low back pain, and use ten different ideas and sets of points on all ten patients.

Acupuncture in a book, or a case study, is a very static thing. Practicing in clinic is anything but static.

I also prescribe herbs, supplements, a cold laser, cupping (rarely), and micro current for local point stimulation. If I have a patient who feels the need for local stimulation, I use a micro current device.

Theory

You will see sometimes I emphasize one theory with a case study. This doesn't mean that I was *only* using one theory for that case, or just one theory for any case. I chose to highlight certain theories in different cases so the reader can hopefully see most if not all theories highlighted at least once.

The theories of Tung and other Distal methods are the "3 jiaos, 12 segments, tissue for tissue, channel relationships, 5 elements, Dao Ma concept, reaction area, images, mirrors, start and end of channels, Chinese clock time, seasonal change, Tung family unique channel/points/ Zang relationships, 5 Zang lines, and clinical experience.

By no means do you need to know all this theory, you can choose to delve into it or keep it as simple as you want. I love to learn all the reasons why, because it helps me make sense of it all, and it also helps me to remember. Also, remember these points work regardless of what theory we use. The points work! Plain and simple.

If learning the theory is too much work, you can just memorize the points, actions and indications. It is up to you. You have to be careful the more intricate we get about theory. There is always some theory that contradicts another theory. It is OK. It is just theory. It is fun. Sometimes we have to let go of the reason why we do something, and just do it.

Point Selection

I have chosen a variety of random cases. I did this to demonstrate as many points as possible. This is not how it is in the clinic. You will use 20% of your points 80% of the time. In my experience, if you know 20-30 Master

Tung points, and are very familiar with them, you would feel very comfortable treating at least 80% of your patients. Yes, it is fun to learn all of them, and you should. However, acupuncture is like a language, there are 500 words that are used all the time. If you are familiar with them, you can get by easily. The Tung system is similar to TCM, the top 20 points can be used to treat most ailments.

Alternating Points

When you do sports training, you will improve faster when you do a variety of exercises. You will get the best results when you continually surprise the body. It is the same with acupuncture. I do not do the same points for every treatment. The body heals faster if we use a variety of points. We can use the same theory, treat the same root, and the same disease, but keep changing points throughout the course of treatment.

Local and Distal

I do not advise using Tung points with local TCM points, because they both via different mechanisms. However, if you are new to Tung acupuncture, it will take some time to learn the system. You have been using TCM since you learned it in school. You do not have to start using all Tung points.

The easiest way to learn this method is to start your treatment with distal points. If you achieve the desired results, then there is no need to continue with local needles. If you failed, then go ahead and treat locally. This is business decision. If you go out of business, you will not be able to practice any medicine, let alone Tung points. As you learn and become more comfortable, you can use more Tung points and fewer local TCM points. Tung points take all the guesswork out, it works right there in front of you and your patient.

Finally

Master Tung used Western medical terminology to explain things, and so have I. When Master Tung was asked why, he replied that Western medicine was more accepted during his time. This is not to disrespect TCM theory. I just choose to communicate in a language that my patients understand.

Master Tung was known for not talking much. When students asked him a question, he would often tell them to observe for themselves. Dr. Tan is also very much like this. When I interned in his clinic, he allowed me to ask just three questions a day.

At that time, he saw around 40-50 patients a day. I would follow him all day and get just three questions. You learn to think for yourself, just as Master Tung advised. I mention this to suggest you also form your own opinions. This book is meant only as a guide, as a starting point. Please continue to research, study, practice, think, fail, try again, read some more, practice, be inquisitive, and challenge yourself!

I have no magic needles and no special potions. I have no ancient Chinese secrets, or privileged information. If I can do this, *anybody can*! Observe for yourself, think, analyze, change, improvise, overcome and adapt. I hope this case study book helps. I hope it is a great starting point in your journey of learning.

CHAPTER ONE

BASICS OF MASTER TUNG THEORY

Ashi Locations (Tender Points)

There is no need to locate Ashi points when treating pain or other ailments. You can treat Ashi locations if you like. However, Tung points do not require a point to be tender. In some cases, I find the Tung point and then look for an Ashi point around it, but it is not necessary. The point will still be effective even if you find it and there is *no* Ashi sensation.

Needle Gauge

You can use any size or brand you like. I use 36 gauge. I know some acupuncturists who use 28 gauge, and or 40 gauge. Any size will work. You do not need to tonify, sedate, rotate, or flick. There is no needling manipulation in the Tung system. Insert your needles and relax. Make sure your needles are not "flopping all over", but you do not need to needle deeply either. The depth of insertion for most points is .25-.50 cun on the arms. The legs are .5-1.5 cun. The fingers and head are around .1-.3 cun

Internal Medicine

Although the focus of this book is pain relief, Master Tung points are equally effective for internal disorders. Most Western patients will only seek acupuncture for pain conditions, so if you are successful at treating pain, you will be trusted to treat other health problems.

Treatment Duration

The cycle of Qi is around 28 minutes. MRI studies have shown that the brain will continue to respond for 28.8 minutes. I have my patients sit or recline for 25-30 minutes.

Number of Needles

We should always try to limit the number of needles we use. However, it is important to not just insert a few needles and assume you have done enough. You should continue to address other affected channels until you get complete pain relief. The goal is to use as few needles as possible, but as many as you need to get results. Get feedback from your patients. Ask where the pain is and treat the remainder of the pain.

Patient Response

You should expect 90-100% pain relief of your patient on the treatment table. In my experience, 85% of patients will get this level of relief. Ten percent have 25-75% pain relief during treatment. Five percent do not get complete relief during treatment.

Some acupuncturists treat patients three times a week. I do not. I see most of my patients once a week, and in some cases twice a week. Of the 100 patients that I treat per week, only 16 of them come twice a week.

I always advise my patients to allow three to four treatments before we can determine if acupuncture will help them. This does not always work. Some patients do not return. Some only get one or two treatments. We expect instant pain relief in most cases. We expect lasting relief, but I always recommend three to four visits over a ten-day period to see how patients respond. After the initial series of treatments, we decide what further treatments are necessary.

Opposite Side Treatment

You will treat most points on the non-affected (opposite) side. If you are in doubt, treat the opposite side. However, there are some points that theoretically could be treated on the same side.

Having Patients Move During Treatment

Insert the needles and ask the patient to move, and see if the pain is still there. Within one to two seconds, you will know if you have gotten it. If they cannot move while on the table, or recreate the pain, treat the pain as if it were present during the treatment. After the treatment, your patient can try to recreate the pain.

Summary

One thing I really like about Master Tung acupuncture is that it is straightforward. Insert the needles, breathe, and heal. That is it! There are no tricks, no magic, and no guessing. It is just easy, safe, effective, reliable, reproducible, consistent, and amazingly effective acupuncture.

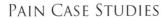
In the realm of ideas everything depends on enthusiasm... in the real world all rests on perseverance.

Johann Wolfgang von Goethe

CHAPTER TWO

CASE STUDIES

LOW BACK AND HIP PAIN IN AN 82-YEAR-OLD MAN

MAIN COMPLAINT

This patient hates acupuncture, mainly because he does not believe in it. However, his daughter, whom I treat for side effects from medications, has had good results, and has since convinced her father to come in.

He is 82 years old, and his complaint is that he cannot walk to his mailbox to the get the mail. He is in constant pain. He has left hip and left lower back pain at L2-5, S1-4. He basically is hurting everywhere, yet he does not care. His sole complaint is not the pain itself, but the fact that he cannot walk to the mailbox. He cannot hear well; therefore, that makes it very challenging to diagnose him correctly. The only request that this patient has is for his back to feel better. Another issue that we have is that he does not want to undress, which makes it difficult to get him onto the treatment table, due to his hearing problem and the pain that he is in.

MERIDIAN INVOLVED /THEORY

He has pain in the lower back at L2-5/S1-4, which radiates further out to the hip and down his left leg onto the BL and GB channels. The pain stops at the BL 40 and GB 34 area.

TREATMENT POINTS

This patient does not want to disrobe, or take his shoes, or socks off. I had him roll up his pants to the knees in order to treat him.

Left side	BL 40 and GB 34 – guide points; I insert BL 40 from the side so that you can use this point when people lie on their backs. These are my *guide points*, and same side treatment points.
Right side	TW 14 LI 15 LU 2 SI 10, and three needles from each of these points; one cun distally from each other. 33.12 22.04 22.05 San Cha San San Cha Yi San Cha Er 22.08 22.09 And modified SI 4 points

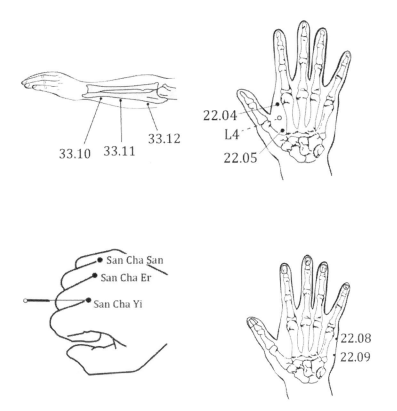

OUTCOME

I like this case because the patient was only in pain when he walked, and of course, he did not have any pain when I treated him. Even though I asked him to walk around in my clinic, he said it would only hurt when he walked to the mailbox. Therefore, the outcome was unknown.

COMMENTS

He informed me that he would not schedule another treatment. Instead, he wanted to wait and determine if the acupuncture had worked. I had no idea if it had, for obvious reasons. He could not hear very well, and he was not in pain during the treatment; therefore, it was impossible to know if I was helping him or not.

The patient was not interested in anything other than getting out of pain. He had been in pain for over 30 years, and of course, nothing thus far had helped. He argued that acupuncture could not help, especially since the needles were not placed where the pain was located.

Now let us fast-forward two weeks. The patient's daughter called in to my office today to schedule her father for treatment again. He has been walking every day since he was treated, and there was no more pain when he walked. He wants to continue treatment for all of his other aches and pains.

This is extremely important, because at times, you have to meet a patient where he is. In this case, if I could not treat the first problem, there is no way he would let me treat his other aches and pains. This is the type of patient that will only believe a procedure is helpful when he gets results.

The treatment that I used was so effective because of the layering, and the use of multiple images. The shoulder, elbow and hand all imaged the lower back.

I treated the BL, KD, and GB, as well as the joint spaces of L5/S1. This also helped us remember to focus on the root. His leg did hurt, but was it just leg pain, or was it a problem with the joint of L2-5/S1-4 that was causing the radiation down his leg? By treating the root and the joint, we were able to stop the pain radiation.

I do not believe I will be able to get all of his pain to go away. He is older, and his age will be a major factor as to why he will not get enough treatments. However, I have promised him that he will at least have a reduction in his pain; he should have at least a 50% reduction in joint pain.

The patient is extremely excited, due to the fact that he has no problem living with 50% less pain. I think we can relieve more pain, but that will take longer and require a little bit of luck. The treatments will fix his main concern, which is the back, leg, and pain radiation, but some of the minor areas might prove to be challenging.

I just received an update. I treated his daughter last night, and she said that her dad is doing great. He is walking to the mailbox every morning. The patient is sleeping better, he is a bit less cantankerous, and he moves much more than he had been. The patient's daughter also informed me that her father is very happy and excited for his two treatments next week. He told her that he has no idea how or why it works, but that it works for him.

Sciatica from Moving Big Equipment

MAIN COMPLAINT

A 47-year-old man has sciatica. He is a machinist, and he walks all day in boots on concrete floors. He also bends a lot, and moves big equipment all day by lifting and dragging.

His back pain is chronic; so much so, that it has now developed into very painful sciatica that radiates down to his toes. He is in constant pain. To give an accurate reading of the pain, his score - when he has a flare-up - is 7 to 8, out of 10.

The pain is primarily on the right side, but the left side also hurts. That pain usually radiates to the right GB and BL channels. At times it radiates down the ST channel. In the last two weeks, the patient has experienced pain radiating down both of his legs. The bilateral pain is intermittent.

MERIDIAN INVOLVED /THEORY

BL, GB, KD, and Du for the back; L3-4-5, S1-2-3-4
ST channels were treated for the times that it radiates to the front.
Degeneration of the joints and muscles, he is just "wearing out," as he says.

POINTS USED

The pain at time of treatment was on the right lower back, and radiating down the ST channel to the knee. It also radiated down the BL channel from BL 40 to BL 67. He could not tell for sure where the pain was coming from, but he thought he felt some of the pain on the GB channel. (This is called compartmental pain syndrome in Western medicine).

There is no pain from the back to the knee on the bladder channel, but there is pain from the knee to the foot. You would think that it is knee pain radiating to the foot, but it is *not*. It originates in the back at L5/S1. In this case, the brain is not telling the patient that his mid-thigh hurts. Hence, it is called compartmental syndrome.

Opposite side	22.04
	22.05
	22.08
	22.09
	33.12
	Gu Ci Yi
	Gu Ci Er
	Gu Ci San
	33.04
	33.05
	33.06 needled from TW meridian down to the PC meridian
Same side	BL 65
	ST 43 (or, 66.05)
	Same side GB 43, or, 66.08 and 66.09

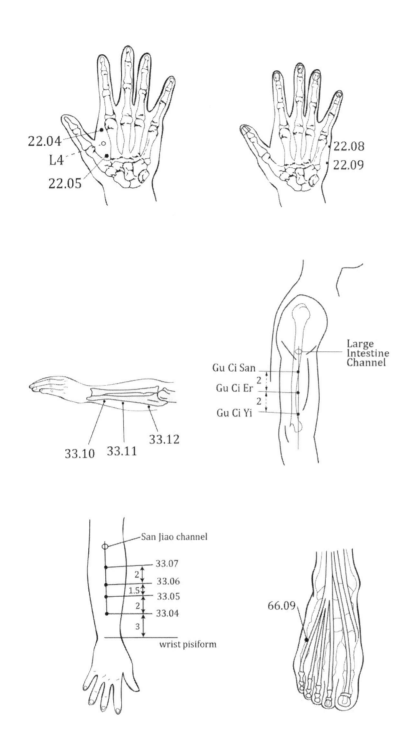

OUTCOME

During our first treatment, his pain has reduced by 50%, and his pain radiated only to the mid-thigh. It had previously radiated to his toes. This is a classic case of when the pain did not go away completely, and this is OK. The patient is happy, and I was happy. Sometimes that is all you can get.

We could have added more needles. However, there were already enough (too many) needles. Could I have chosen better points, or applied a different theory in order to receive a better outcome? Perhaps, but this is learning from experience. We are all learning, every day. That is why I always make it a point to stress the importance of reading books, and studying. However, you learn the most from treating patients. Books can explain theory, but we need to prove that theory in real life.

I have scheduled this patient for two treatments a week, over the next four weeks. This will be a difficult case, due to the requirements of his job. He is 6'1" tall, and tall men typically have back problems. His pain has been chronic for 20 years now, but at this point in his life, it has become too painful to endure, but the other issue is that he cannot stop working, and apparently finding another job is not an option. As we continue treatments, he will continue to re-injure his back. After our first treatment using distal points, he was shocked at how much better he felt. He is now on board, as he says. The patient informed me that he cannot take pain medications because he works around heavy machinery.

COMMENTS

We can easily make sciatica very complicated. You just have to look at *all* the Tung points that are indicated *just for sciatic* pain. There so many, which include:

11.11-12
22.04-5-6-7-8-9
33.04-5-6-7-8-9-12
44.01-2-3, 14-15-16,

55.04-5
66.01-13-14-15
77.-01-2-3-4-5-6-7-27
88.12-13-14-17-18-19
1010.-1-2-3-4-21-22-24-25
San Cha San, San Cha Yi, San Cha Er

These points are *just for sciatica*. They are not meant to be used for low back pain, or the other 50 complaints related to the back. I am sure there are more points. However, these are just the points that I can think of off of the top of my head. We *could* make it very complicated, but we should try to keep it as simple as possible.

Points 22.04 and 22.05, which is the Ling Gu and Da Bai combination, are a very reliable treatment.

Points 22.08 and 22.09 are great for low back pain and kidney/age related pain, due to the reaction area of the kidney. The SI channel gets the BL channel. The image is perfect for sciatica as well.

We need multiple images. We need to layer, expand, and be redundant with our images. Therefore, I added in 33.12, which is good for S1-4 and coccyx pain.

With Gu Ci Yi, Gu Ci Er, Gu Ci San, we are now on the LI channel, and the reaction area of the Du/spine. We are tapping the bone with these points so that we also treat bone problems. The image of the upper arm can be the reverse image of the lower back. LI fixes Kidney.

I needled TW 33.04, 33.05, 33.06 because the TW will treat the GB, and needling deep from the TW to the PC will treat the radiation down the ST channel. I did not want to add any more points. It is OK to needle through to the other channels. An example is needling from KD to BL, and even ST to BL. Another option is the TW to PC, or SI over to HT. You can even needle from the plantar side 66.03 and 66.04, down to 55.01, which is on the bottom of the foot (or the hand, Ling Gu, Da Bai over to 22.01 and 22.02)

After this, we will need to guide our treatment to where we want it to go. So we chose BL 65, or GB 43 and ST 43, or respective Tung points. I like using 66.08 and 66.09 because not only does it guide the treatment to the GB channel, but 66.08 and 66.09 are also indicated for general bone swelling, as well as random aches and pains.

The patient was very happy that the pain radiating down his ST channel was completely gone, and his back no longer hurt. He said he could still feel some twinges of pain, but overall, he was excited and happy about his treatment.

Remember to always keep it simple, and let the body do all of the thinking. Watch your channels, look at your underlying pathology, look at the micro of the patient, and then expand back in order to see the big picture. Use your points to treat the whole system, but then you should also have some points that specifically treat the root of the pain in the L5/S1 area. See the yin and yang, but do not forget the yang within the yin, and the yin within the yang. We treated the branch, which was his pain, but we also treated his root, which was age-related degeneration of bones/kidney/muscles and tendons. Expand your images. Always be redundant in your images, channels, and theories.

SHOULDER PAIN IN A MASSAGE THERAPIST

MAIN COMPLAINT

A 41-year-old woman suffered from right side shoulder pain, as well as her supraspinatus, posterior deltoid, serratus anterior, teres minor and major – also on the right side.

I have been treating this patient on and off for over three years now. She is a massage therapist, right handed, and about every six-to-nine months, she will come in for two-to-three visits in order to keep her shoulder healthy. Her pain is always in the right shoulder. It is the result of an old injury she had when she was 32. Her pain now just flares up from time-to-time because of all the bodywork that she does.

MERIDIAN INVOLVED /THEORY

All the meridians in the shoulder are affected. Most of the pain is in the posterior shoulder, and although we think of this as the SI channel, it is really the tendon from the supraspinatus that hooks into the posterior deltoid. The supraspinatus is controlled by the TW channel; however, you can also view it as the SI (as per TCM as well). It is worth noting that when treating pain, you will find that it works better if you treat the TW using the relationship of the muscle tendino channels. (the Jing Jin relationships)

The patient's trapezius is a bit involved, which is controlled by the BL and GB channels. The primary location of pain is on the lateral side of the chest, serratus anterior, armpit, teres minor, and major. The TW, SI, and GB channels control all these muscles. We can take it a step further and say that her sub scapular muscles are involved. The LI channel controls them.

She has long-term inflammation, chronic pain, swelling, blood stagnation, muscle, ligament, and tendon problems.

TREATMENT POINTS

This patient DOES NOT LIKE NEEDLES!

Same side hand	San Cha San 33.16
Opposite hand	Fan Hou Jue 44.06
Opposite leg	77.18 77.20 77.24 77.25
Same leg	77.09

OUTCOME

Every time the patient comes in, she does well; it takes 2-3 treatments to get her 100% out of pain. She is scheduled for Monday and Thursday of next week, at which point I will release her again. If she would commit to a longer course of treatment, she would completely heal, but she is happy with getting two-to-three treatments every six-to-nine months.

The patient always feels a thick, achy, dull pain in her shoulder. She also reports feeling restricted in her movement. After her treatment, she feels relieved, lighter, and is in less pain, with an improved range of motion.

COMMENTS

I continually default to Fan Hou Jue, and 77.09, as my best choice for shoulder points. These two points are mostly irrespective of channel selection. It does not matter where the pain is, these points will typically fix it all.

I use San Cha San as my guide point, since a lot of her pain is on her supraspinatus - that is where her pain originates.

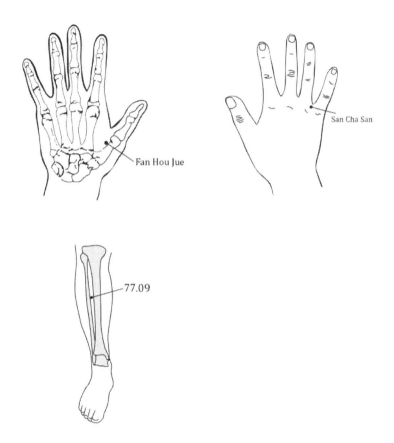

I use 33.16 here as a distal point that is almost local – it is LU 5. I like this point because part of her pain is on the Tai Yin meridian, plus 33.16/LU 5 is near a big tendon. Treating a big tendon fixes tendon issues. The same side LU treats the LU channel in her shoulder; the lower arm will treat the upper arm.

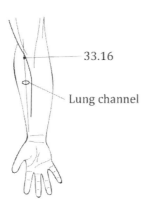

On the opposite arm, point 44.06, is in the deltoid. The healthy arm can treat the sick arm. It is also in thick muscles. We are treating the earth, the spleen, and muscles. All these things are out of balance with her constitution. In addition to that, this is the reaction area of the cardiac nerve, which makes it very good for blood flow.

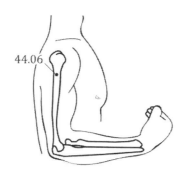

The opposite leg, 77.18, is the shoulder. It is true that the entire arm can be on half of the leg. Here, the knee is the shoulder. This point is also a good choice due to the fact that the SP will treat the SI channel. You would treat the posterior shoulder via the SI channel, according to TCM theory. The SP channel also treats the TW, which is the muscle that is actually causing the pain. The supraspinatus is used according to the muscle tendino channels, which are the channels we should be treating with pain.

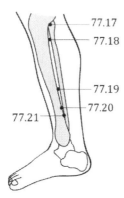

In my experience, with most cases of true frozen shoulder, the patient will not be able to magically raise her arm when you needle 77.18. It can happen, and it sometimes does work out that way, but it is the exception, rather than the rule. This is when the shoulder problem fits the medical definition of frozen shoulder.

Do not think that all of your frozen shoulder patients will get complete relief with one or two needles. You will be able to help them, and in some cases, have a complete resolution of the problem; however, it is more difficult to treat in most cases.

Point 77.20 is the image of the shoulder on the eighth of the leg. Therefore, the whole arm is put on a quarter of the leg. We have different images on one leg. It is also the reaction area of the four limbs, so it is great for shoulder and limb pain.

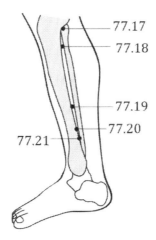

Points 77.24 and 77.25 are remarkable for shoulder pain. We are using different meridians here, which is good, and now we have half the arm on the leg. The GB will treat the TW channel, and the GB channel will treat the armpit. It also treats HT 1-2-3 area using the Zang Fu Bei Tong theory. Here, the image of the shoulder is the whole arm, and it fits on a quarter of the leg. It is an image within an image.

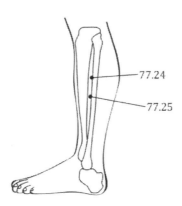

Do I use ST 41 and LV 4? Yes, but on this patient it is a bit too painful. This is one reason I love understanding the theories behind the points. If you just memorize points, you will not be as effective; instead, you will be controlled, and stuck. In the end, you will be just a cook, and a follower.

To be a true chef in the kitchen, you must understand flavors, smells, temperature, and tastes. As a chef in acupuncture, you must know the *theory*. Using theory, you can apply it in a fluid motion. This is the magic of acupuncture, learning to be fluid with your stuck patient.

Could I use the knuckles of the hand to treat the shoulder? Yes, this is a good image and many people use it. The knuckles, on opposite sides of the hand, treat the shoulder, but this patient hates the knuckle points.

Knowing the indication of points is good, but understanding theory is the *key*. If you apply the theory, the points will appear. If you look for the points without using the theory, then they will be hidden.

Rib Pain from a Car Accident

MAIN COMPLAINT

A 47-year-old woman was in a car accident over a year ago. Her lung collapsed during the accident, and she almost died from multiple traumatic injuries. Her ribs were broken on the left side. The affected area was the intercostal spaces 6-7-8. The emergency technician had to insert a breathing tube due to her collapsed lung; it was placed in the location of her broken ribs. This no doubt saved her life, but because of the tube insertion, she now has pain in that area.

The car accident occurred approximately 14 months ago. The patient still has tremendous pain in the area where her ribs were broken, as well as the area into which the breathing tube was inserted. She is in constant pain, which ranges from 4-7/10, depending on what she is doing. She has taken pain medications, physical therapy, and now is doing acupuncture.

I treated this patient over three years ago for random aches and pains, with a complete resolution of her symptoms. She has come back, because she had success with her previous ailment. She is also frustrated, because she has still not recovered from her accident.

MERIDIAN INVOLVED /THEORY

The ST, SP, and GB meridians all run through the ribs.
The ribs have a history of trauma, inflammation, irritation, Qi and blood stagnation, phlegm, and dampness.

There is residual trauma, and the area where the breathing tube was inserted into the ribs is not healing.

TREATMENT POINTS

Opposite arm/leg	33.04 33.05 33.06 alternated each treatment with 33.08 and 33.09 11.07 and 77.26 --alternated each treatment with 77.05, 77.06, 77.07 with 77.26
Same side	88.20 88.21 88.22 88.25 88.17 88.18 88.19

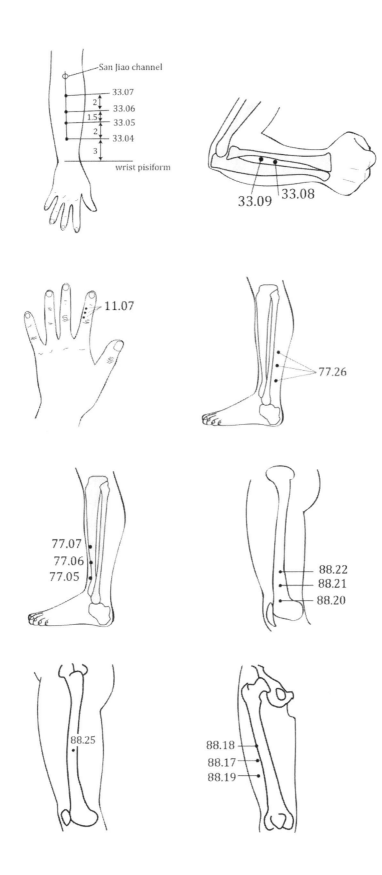

OUTCOME

During treatment, she reported that she no longer had pain in her ribs. Sometimes it hurts to breathe, but it is only occasionally, not every breath. We continue to treat her one session per week. I advised her that it will take four to eight treatments to completely heal, and after treatment, she will be able to breathe with no pain. She has had three treatments at the time of this case study.

During each treatment, her pain is resolved and stays away for approximately 4-7 days. When the pain comes back, it is less intense. The pain is more localized, affecting a smaller area. The patient is also breathing better.

COMMENTS

Every time I treated this patient, her pain was relieved, and her breathing improved. The tissue was intact, but it had chronic swelling, inflammation, trauma, as well as blood/Qi/phlegm stagnation in her ribs.

I believe I could have also treated the lung function in order to improve breathing, but on this patient, it did not seem appropriate. I chose to focus on the rib pain, stagnation, swelling, and trauma. The following points also treat systemic inflammation, swelling, phlegm, Qi, and blood stagnation.

Points 33.04, 33.05, 33.06 are on the lower arm. The hand images the head. The lower arm images the upper part of the torso. The belly button images the elbow. Therefore, the mid lower arm to the wrist represents the rib cage area. Points 33.04, 33.05, 33.06 are indicated for rib pain, heart issues, and chest pain. The points are on the TW channel and they treat the GB and SP channels that run through her chest. The TW also is imperative for helping the mesenteric artery system, which is responsible for much of the inflammation that is around the thoracic cavity.

I especially like the points 33.08 and 33.09, because they are .5 cun lateral to the TW channel, and are actually on top of the ulna. When we needle these points, we are activating the TW and SI channels, because we are between the TW and SI channels. More importantly, we are also treating *bone*. The ribs are damaged. We need to needle bone to heal them. These two points tap the bone.

Points 88.20, 88.21, 88.22, 88.25 are treated on the same side due to the fact that the same side GB treats the GB. One way we can image this is to find the ribs and see where they intersect on the arm. The ribs are on the same line, just above the elbow. The elbow is the knee. Therefore, we needle just above the knee, on the correct channel.

Points 88.17, 88.18, 88.19 are indicated for rib pain, breathing, and lung issues such as allergies. In this case, we were using them for rib pain and lung/breathing issues. These points run between the ST and GB channels, and thus will treat both ST and GB. Both of these channels run through the painful area. These points are on the Five Zang line of the lung, thus they will treat lung issues/breathing issues; it is the image of the lungs and ribs. The upper thigh is the upper chest area. These are probably some of the top 5-10 points used all of the time in Tung acupuncture. These points are very valuable for treatments.

The Three Weights

Points 11.07 and 77.05, 77.06, 77.07 are both called *the three weights*. The most popular points, referred to as the three weights, are the points 77.05, 77.06, 77.07, but the three-point unit 11.07 is called the finger three weights. They have the same indications. The leg points, 77.05, 77.06, 77.07 are stronger and more effective. However, the finger points 11.07 are great for rib pain.

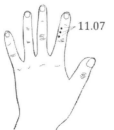
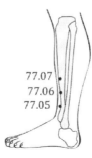

The three-point unit, 77.26, is more popular for neck pain. It is on the BL channel. The lower leg images the upper neck. The most important thing about these points is that they are the reaction area for the rib cage. This Dao Ma is very important and very effective for rib pain.

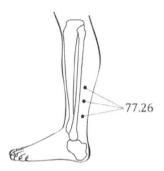

It will take some time to resolve this patient's pain completely. I advised her she will need between 45-60 days to resolve the problem she has had for 18 months. When she is in pain, we are able to resolve it immediately on the treatment table.

Random Walk-In Patients

I often have people walk in off the street to check my office out. I have three treatment rooms, along with an herb room, an office, a bathroom, and a waiting room. I have one couch, and two chairs to sit and relax in while in the clinic.

People often just walk in and say that they are in pain and that they need help. I can usually get people scheduled within 48 hours, but my treatment rooms are usually full, or will be soon. Therefore, it makes it nearly impossible for me to treat people who walk in with no appointment.

What I usually do with walk-in patients is I have them sign a quick waiver. I ask them where their pain is, and tell them I can insert two to three needles while they sit for ten minutes. I want to relieve their pain immediately. I tell them they might be pain free for 24-48 hours. This will give me a chance to fit them into my regular appointment schedule, so that I can get to the root of their problems.

In the last three weeks, I have had four of these walk-in patients. Since I have not done a full intake on these people, the only information I have is what I can gather from what they tell me, or what I can guess from experience. I do not take the pulse, and I do not look at the tongue. I have them sit down and tell me what their main problem is. I then insert two to three needles. This whole process usually takes less than three minutes. This is the amount of time that I have to spend with these people, because I am going from room to room treating my scheduled patients.

The following are three case studies from these walk-in patients.

Back Pain Walk-In

A middle-aged woman walked in with x-rays in her hand and started complaining of back pain. She did not bother to say hello or ask for an appointment. She just started talking to me as I walked out of a treatment room. My wife works the front office, but was away from the office on that particular day. As I walked out, the woman started talking to me about her back pain, and where it was that she hurt. She wanted to be seen immediately.

After I calmed her down, and she signed a waiver, I scheduled her for the following week. It was Friday and the soonest I could see her was Tuesday. I did not want to send her home to spend the weekend in pain. I also did not want her to feel I had not listened to, or cared for her.

I do not charge for these types of treatments. It is "put up or shut up" time for them. It is where the rubber meets the road. It is also where patients, who have no idea about acupuncture, who do not believe in it, are upset, in severe pain, or angry and they want to be out of pain *right now*.

These patients do not disrobe. I do not have them take off their shoes or socks. I typically treat the lower leg. I often just treat their hands, and lower arms. Another option is to treat their face and head, because that area is also exposed.

This patient had low back pain. Her x-rays confirmed this. Her verbal assault of me as I walked out of the treatment room confirmed that what she had been doing to treat her pain was not working. She needed help.

I treated:

Opposite side	San Cha San San Cha Er San Cha Yi Ling Gu
Same side	1010.25 Ear Shen Men Ear back points Ear Point Zero

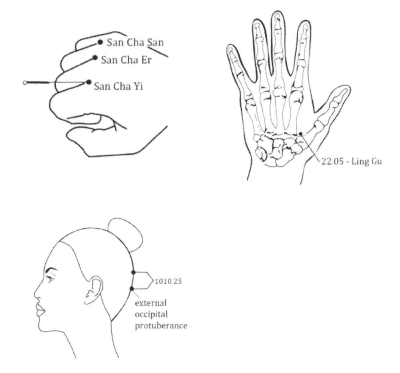

The points in the ear were used to calm her down. Ear Shen Men, point zero, and back pain points on the ear are very effective to treat low back pain. Master Tung has a few points on the ear, but not for these indications.

45

San Cha Yi, San Cha Er, and San Cha San cover the whole low back, low hip, and low gluteal area. Point 1010.25 is great for L2-5/S1-2 pain.

I had her sit for ten minutes. I left her to treat my next patient and when I came out, she was calm. She had 70% less pain. She had put down her x-rays, and was sitting on the couch, relaxing. She was kinder, slower, softer, and much more amicable.

Her pain was reduced and she now had hope. Hope is very powerful. As long as your patients have hope, they can usually get better. People with no hope are lost.

Headache Walk-In

A few days later, another person walked into my office. She would not schedule until she was able to "vet" me about who I was, and how long I had been practicing.

I told her I was busy and was willing to make an appointment, and we could go over all this then. She hesitated, then I asked her if she was a "betting" woman. I said "I bet you if you give me ten minutes and one needle, we can reduce your headache (her main complaint) by at least fifty percent."

She consented and I inserted 22.04, Da Bai. I had her breathe and slow down. She then reported her headache was still there, however "the pain, the piercing pain in my head has been greatly reduced." I explained that this was 1% of what Chinese medicine could do for her. I suggested she schedule a new patient appointment so we could chat about her whole health history.

One point	22.04, Da Bai

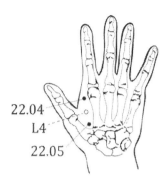

Twisted Ankle Walk-In

This last week a person showed up with a twisted ankle. She was a middle-aged female who limped into my office and told me she had twisted her ankle when she was horseback riding. She did not have time to talk to me and was curious about going to the emergency room.

Many people in my community come to my clinic before going to the emergency room. They want my opinion, and my advice. That is what my acupuncture clinic has become; it is viewed as a trusted place of appropriate medical care. I do not, and cannot, treat many of the people who walk-in, but I always suggest who they should see or where they need to go for care.

They get an honest, no BS opinion of what, and how, they should proceed. My advice is not affected by my personal financial gain. Many practitioners rarely discuss options outside of their scope of practice. In my opinion, it is our duty to discuss any and all health options, whether or not we provide that care.

In this case, I told her that she should go to the emergency room for an x-ray, and possible MRI to check for a break in her ankle. We could do acupuncture, and if she felt better for longer than four hours, this would be an indication that her bone was not broken. With broken bones and tumors, the pain could be relieved. If it does get better, it only stays better for less than four hours. After four hours, the pain will return.

I inserted Xiao Jie. It is on the palm of the hand. It starts at the base of the first metacarpal joint, and goes superficially to PC 7. It's best for medial ankle pain, but it is so effective that it will treat the entire ankle.

One point	Xiao Jie

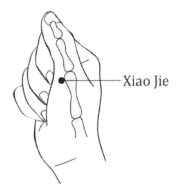

Xiao Jie

The patient had an 85% reduction in pain with that one needle. I had her rest for 15 minutes, and then I told her to either go straight to the emergency room, or wait four hours and see if the pain came back.

She called later that night and thanked me for a few things. She appreciated that I treated her immediately, and free of charge. She was grateful for the pain relief, and she appreciated the fact that I told her to go to the emergency room.

Her pain did return later that evening. It took longer than four hours, but her pain did come back. She went to the emergency room and sure enough, she had a small stress fracture. She is currently in a cast and says she will call to schedule an appointment with me when her cast comes off.

I do not think she will call, and I am sure I could have pushed her harder to schedule. This type of practice is taught in some practice management programs. However, I do not operate like that. If she wants to come in, she can; if she does not, that is fine as well.

I do not like scripts, and I do not like locking the patient down with contracts for multiple treatments. It just felt wonderful to help a person in pain.

The reason I am using this case as an example is to highlight the point, Xiao Jie. It is an amazing point for ankle pain. I also wanted to show how sometimes, no matter how powerful our points are, we cannot solve all health problems. We do our best, are honest, and work hard, but sometimes, it is out of our hands.

Dizziness Walk-In

One walk-in patient that came into my office this week was dizzy. Dizzy patients can be scary. A lot of dangerous things can cause dizziness, and I do not suggest treating them. I had treated this woman before. I checked her blood pressure and it was only 140/90, which is high, but not dangerous. She signed a waiver saying that after the treatment she would go to the emergency room, regardless of the acupuncture treatment outcome.

I treated 77.05, 77.06, 77.07 on the left side, and LI 11 on the right. I had her sit for 10 minutes. When I returned, her dizziness was 50% relieved. I added 1010.01, 1010.05, and 1010.06. When I returned 10 minutes later, she reported that 90% of her dizziness was gone.

Left side	77.05
	77.06
	77.07
Right side	LI 11
	1010.01
	1010.05
	1010.06

LI 11, via the 12 segments, is the head; it helps with head issues. It is also Yang Ming, so it has a lot of Qi and blood.

49

Points 1010.01, 1010.05, 1010.06 are the reaction area of the brain. They are very important for brain issues, but she also had an element of stress, and these points helped to calm her down.

Points 77.05, 77.06, 77.07 are indicated for Meniere's disease, dizziness, GB wind, Qi stagnation, masses, systemic Qi and blood stagnation, as well as all sorts of issues. These are very effective points.

Again, I do not suggest treating dizzy people when they come in. However, in her case, I made a calculated guess, took a risk, and I was lucky. I normally send people like this straight to the emergency room.

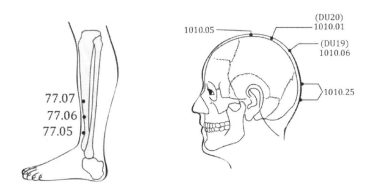

IT Band Pain in a Runner

MAIN COMPLAINT

A 27-year-old man had pain on his right side, on the IT band, from the hip to the knee, on the GB channel. After running all weekend, his hip hurts when he walks or bends over. He walked in my office, limping from the pain.

MERIDIAN INVOLVED /THEORY

The GB channel along the IT band is an acute attack. Since it is so "new," it should resolve very quickly. Do not over complicate things.

TREATMENT POINTS

I used a homologous relationship, I treated the shoulder, and walked points down the arm to the elbow.

My guide point was 77.27. This treatment was repeated three times total for a complete recovery.

OUTCOME

The patient felt complete relief as he lay on the treatment table, when I treated the homologous opposite shoulder. I needled down the TW channel on the arm in order to fix the leg. I inserted TW 14, and then I inserted five needles, equally spaced, down the TW channel to TW 10.

I had the patient flex his leg, bending it and straightening it while the needles were in. He was able to find painful points when he palpated himself prior to the needle insertion. I asked him to go back to those painful areas and palpate again; he was unable to locate the painful areas.

Same side, right side	77.27 – guide point
Opposite side	TW 14, plus five needles equally spaced down the TW channel, to TW 10.

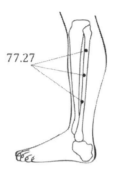

77.27

COMMENTS

This is a great example of *not over thinking* the issue. He had a common inflammation and basic trauma to his IT band. I suspect it was already injured, and his last long run was just enough to push his body over the limit, to the point that he was not able to recover. There was no need to diagnose him for an hour, and go through ten questions, ultimately making things very complicated.

If I had wanted to do a complete diagnosis, I might come to the conclusion that this pain was an indication of an underlying pathology. However, in this case, I thought it was simple pain from injury or overuse. The key point here is that I treated the attachment of the IT band, at the head of the femur.

This homologous attachment of the IT band at the head of the femur is at TW 14, where the triceps attaches to the humerus. The other key point is that the pain is on the lateral side of the leg; however, the lateral side of the arm is the Yang Ming channel. The TW channel is on the posterior arm. Make sure you are clear on the correct image. The posterior arm on the TW channel corresponds to the lateral GB channel IT band.

If the patient had still been in pain after inserting five needles, I would have checked for Ashi points, or a "key hole," in order to get the last bit of pain that I missed.

I used 77.27 on the same side. This point is indicated for trauma, and Qi and blood stagnation. I also like it because it not only acts as a guide point, where the lower leg will treat the upper leg, but it is a great way to treat the upper leg.

You might ask if you could also treat the lower arm, TW 4, TW 5, TW 6, TW 7, and TW 8, for the same issue. San Cha San treats the lower leg, and it is great for leg pain. Points 33.04, 33.05, 33.06, 33.08, 33.09 are all great for leg pain. Yes, we can reverse the image so the lower arm treats the upper leg. Yes, it works, and yes, it is great, if you *do not* have access to the upper arm. However, one of the most consistently, effective ways to treat limb pain is using a homologous relationship. This is why I default to this type of treatment. What looks more like the femur and IT band? The lower arm with the radius and ulna? Or the upper arm with the humerus?

You will also find that the homologous relationship is a very reliable and consistent way to treat. This is the same idea as Tung theory of "Name Pairs", such as Lung hand Tai Yin treats leg Tai Yin Spleen. It is also the same as Dr. Tan System One. These are very effective treatment theories. This is by the far the best way to treat limb pain, System One.

All the systems work. All the theories and images work. But the most reliable, and most effective, is *Name Pairs/System One* for limb pain. The homologous relationships are undeniable.

FOLLOW UP

This case is the same issue with a different patient. The other patient was a Western nurse, who had the same exact pain last week, at the same exact location. This time we treated the exact same points. Her pain was 100% relieved on the table. That was Monday. I treated her again on Thursday, and she said that her pain was gone until Thursday morning, but she woke up and 75% of her pain had returned. To me, this was great; to her, I do not think she was as excited. I treated her again on Thursday. She again had 100% pain relief on the treatment table. I advised her that we would need to do two more treatments the following week and reevaluate her.

I advised her that the problem should be resolved by the next week, or the following week. The pain would come back, but it would be less intense. It would also not cover such a large area, it would be less sharp, and she would have a better range of motion. I thought things were going well. However, today I received a message that she had a cortisone shot on Friday, and she wants to cancel her appointments for next week.

What does this tell us? The treatments were successful. However, something was not right for her. It could have been me, the clinic, how I explained things, or any number of things. She needed a different type of medicine. I doubt she will be back. Will she think that acupuncture helped? Probably not.

This is why I tell my patients that I do not do magic! If it were magic, I could treat you one time and that would be all you needed. This is where education and millions of intangibles come into play. Every case is a chance to learn and grow for all of us.

TMJ, Headache, and Pain All Over

MAIN COMPLAINT

A 26-year-old woman has TMJ on the left side, bilateral neck pain, and shooting pains on her arms and legs. She has migraines with her cycle, and appears stressed. She is a stay-at-home mom, and jewelry maker. She loves her life. She is not depressed and she is in a good relationship. She has seen a medical doctor, and all test results are normal. Her doctor prescribed an anti-anxiety drug, and an anti-depressant.

She is not getting relief with Western medicine, so has decided to try acupuncture. After talking with her for about an hour, we have decided to do a quick acupuncture treatment.

Her main complaints are the TMJ on the left side, her headache, and systemic pain.

Points 77.22, 77.23 were inserted on the opposite side. She had a strong Qi sensation. It is not always necessary, but in this case, she did. I then asked her where her pain was. She said her facial pain was gone, but there was some pain remaining at SI 18, just below her eye. I inserted 66.04 on the opposite side. I asked her again where her pain was. She said it was gone. She still had some pain around GB 2. She also had tenderness in her whole body.

I inserted GB 31, or 88.25, on the same side, her left side. Her ear pain was relieved, and her whole body relaxed. Her neck became less tense, and her arms and legs no longer hurt.

POINTS USED

Opposite side, right	77.22 77.23 66.04
Same side, left	GB 31 or 88.25
Right side	22.05, Ling Gu

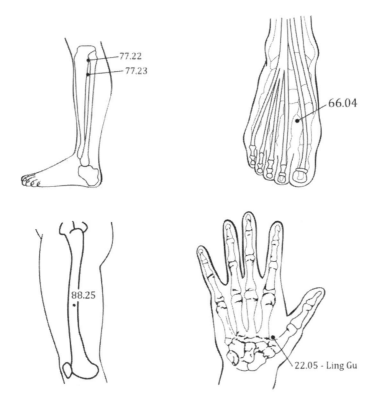

After this, I added 22.05 on the opposite side, for her headaches. Even though 77.22, 77.23 and 88.25, and even 66.04 already covered this. In addition, Ling Gu, 22.05, was added for her other miscellaneous pain, such as low back pain and headaches. This point also moves Qi and blood, treats anemia, regulates her menstrual cycle, relieves stress, and relieves lower leg pain.

This patient is very typical of those in my community. Most residents have never had acupuncture. She is very distrustful of alternative medicine. Western medicine has told her that there is nothing wrong with her. She is tired, stressed, and in pain. She needs help, and she needs an explanation.

To treat a few points, and show her how she really can heal is very powerful for her. She has no insurance, but she has already committed to the next four weeks of care, coming into my office twice a week. This is the power of Tung points in action. Her whole constitution changes in a few minutes after the needles are inserted.

This is an example of how powerful 88.25 is. It is a great point for insomnia, stress, four limb pain, headaches, TMJ, and face pain. It also treats arm pain, and wind issues. The GB channel treats the LV and HT channels. The GB is also bone, per the Ling Shu. There are so many theories to explain this point. Just one point can shift a whole treatment at times.

Points 77.22 and 77.23 are the image of the face. They treat both the ST and GB channels, since they are located between them. It is the reaction area of the teeth. They are very important points for face issues, TMJ, trigeminal neuralgia, and headaches.

Point 66.04, on the LV channel, was used to treat the SI 18 area. The image and channel match up.

As the patient walked out, she remarked that her shoulder and neck felt better (88.25); her low back and legs felt better (22.05); and her face and TMJ were also better (77.22, 77.23, 88.25).

The most powerful statement about this treatment was made when the patient was leaving. She said "Thank you. I have hope again that I can be healthy. Thank you for showing me that this medicine can work." There is power in being able to help the patient by resolving the pain instantly. You do not have to convince her that she will be better over time. Hope is very powerful.

FOLLOW UP

This patient had just one treatment, which lasted only ten minutes. Her first full treatment is scheduled for next week. I received an e-mail this weekend, prior to her full treatment, that she was very thankful that I treated her that first day. The first time a patient comes to my clinic, I do not usually treat them, unless they are in pain. I usually just talk and see if they would like to proceed with 2-3 treatments of acupuncture. She reported that since her ten-minute session on Wednesday, her TMJ had not woken her up at all during the night. Also, her neck and shoulder felt looser. She is excited to come in next week.

I did not charge this patient for her treatment. The reason for this is because we should always put the health of our patients before our money and personal wants. We are here to serve. However, serving and not being paid will not work; therefore, we need to charge people. We should be paid well for our medical skills. Yet, by giving this free treatment (she had no money at the time), I will probably get ten new patients.

The patient wins, she feels better, and is happy. We win because we are helping people for free and that is good Karma. It will grow your practice very fast. I am not saying to give away all treatments for free, I am saying be nice to people and help them out. I had already made enough money for the day, and it was time to give to others. I firmly believe that if you are not helping others with your life, you are wasting your time.

Groin Strain Pain

MAIN COMPLAINT

A 38-year-old man had prostatitis from lifting a heavy lawnmower into his truck. He strained his lower groin muscles, and over time developed an infection in his prostate. This was treated with antibiotics; however, even after multiple courses of antibiotics, his pain remained. The pain was described as a dull, achy pain. It occurred on the pressure of a bowel movement, urination, and sex. The pain extended into the testicles. He described most of this pain as a "dull ache inside."

There were no signs of tissue tears, or a continued infection. His medical doctors were clueless as to why he was still in pain. The pain occurred many times throughout the day. It came and went, depending on what, if any, exercises he was doing. It hurt to lie on the treatment table, because lying on his back increased the pressure in the painful area.

His Western doctor believed that the bacteria became resistant to the drugs. There was also a chance that there was a pocket of infection that the antibiotics just could not treat.

MERIDIAN INVOLVED /THEORY

The affected meridians were the Ren, Du, LV and possibly the KD and BL.

A common theory in Tung acupuncture is that according to five element theory, the spleen (earth) will control, or treat, the kidney (water.)

A very important image is the face for the groin area. The fingers and toes represent the groin area.

The theory is that the start of the channel treats the end of channel, and vice versa.

TREATMENT POINTS

Bilateral	BL 2 1010.09 1010.10 1010.11
Other	Ren 24 Du 26 1010.01 (Du 20)
Opposite hand	11.01 11.02 11.03 11.04 33.01 33.02 33.03
Same side	LV 1 66.03 66.04 66.01 77.18 77.19 77.21

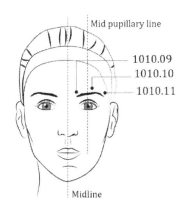

Mid pupillary line

1010.09
1010.10
1010.11

Midline

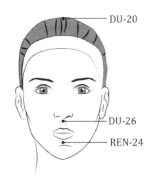

DU-20

DU-26

REN-24

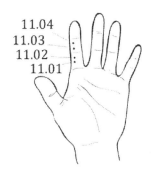

11.04
11.03
11.02
11.01

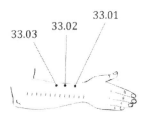

33.03 33.02 33.01

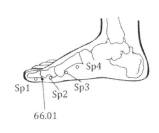

Sp4

Sp1 Sp3
Sp2

66.01

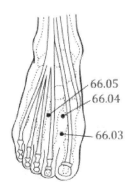

66.05
66.04

66.03

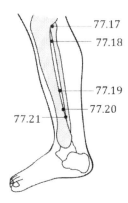

77.17
77.18

77.19
77.20
77.21

After seven treatments using the points above, my new treatment points were:

| Same side | Replaced 77.18, 77.19, and 77.21 with 88.12, 88.13, and 88.14

Replaced 66.01 with 66.02 |
|---|---|
| Bilateral | Replaced 1010.09, 1010.10, and 1010.11 with 1010.21 and 1010.22 |

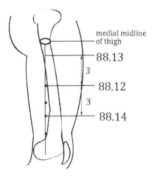

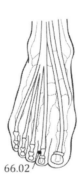

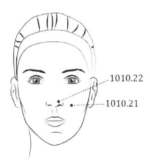

I chose my points according to how he was feeling for each treatment. Other than the points listed as replaced, I used the points every time. There are no substitutes for those points in this case.

OUTCOME

After the first treatment, the patient said the "deep, dull ache was gone." Initially, he was uncomfortable lying on the table, but after the insertion of BL 2 bilaterally, combined with Ren 24 and Du 26, his pain was gone. I continued to address all aspects of the pain by adding points to cover his prostate, bladder, ureters, urethra, penis, and testicles. The pain had been moving through his groin area, although it appeared that the root of the pain was the prostate. I continued to see him six more times and his pain never returned. I saw him twice a week for two weeks, and then once a week for two weeks.

COMMENTS

This case in interesting, because he had gone to a nationally known prostate clinic. His medical doctor was concerned about the pain, but also a possible lingering infection. He had taken a variety of antibiotic cocktails. It was only after he had exhausted all possible options at this prostate clinic, that he returned to Oregon and eventually came to see me.

He had run out of options, so it was time to try acupuncture. He decided acupuncture was a better option than no option. It must be said here as well, this patient hesitated for a month to come see me because he believed I would be putting needles in his penis/prostate area, since that is where he was experiencing pain.

At our initial intake, he was so happy and relieved that all the needles were distal. It was at this time that he mentioned that was one of the biggest reasons why he had not scheduled an appointment for a treatment.

The Liver points are necessary, since the liver meridian encircles the genitals. The foot images the groin, the LV meridian treats the LV.

The LI meridian is often used for sexual health in men and women. The reason for this is that the LI meridian treats the KD, LV, and ST meridians. All these meridians run through the groin. Again, the fingers image the genitals. That is why the points 11.01, 11.02, 11.03, and 11.04 are so great for groin pain.

The eyes image the prostate and testicles.

Ren 24 and Du 26 are the end of the channels, thus they treat the start of the channels, Ren 1 and Du 1.

The point 1010.22 not only images the penis, but it is also useful to treat all pain caused by Qi stagnation. It also treats the spleen/dampness and thus helps with inflammation, via the reaction area.

The point 1010.21 is used to treat all pain caused by blood stagnation. These two points together are wonderful for systemic Qi and blood stagnation causing pain.

One usually thinks of 66.02 for female gynecological problems, but you can use it very effectively for male genital problems as well. The ST channel treats the ST; the foot images the groin area.

Point 66.01 is at the end of the foot, and thus images the groin. The SP meridian will treat the SP, and the ST meridians.

The three emperors, (77.18, 77.19, 77.21), are very effective for all male or female sexual health. They do not treat anything in particular, other than systemic earth fixing water issues. We need to "astringe" and "control," which is why they are used. We needed to control and astringe the inflammation and infection (if any).

FOLLOW UP

This patient called me last week. When he first called, I assumed he was calling about his prostate problem. I apologized that the problem had come back and wanted to try other treatment options. He said he had fallen off his ladder and had back pain. His groin was great. He made an appointment for the following week.

This case shows how we should all work together. Western medical doctors should work with Eastern medicine practitioners. There is no way I could have helped him when he had a resistant strain of bacteria in his prostate. His pain was too intense. He needed painkillers and the infection was too strong for herbs.

After Western medicine fixed the first part of his problem, they were not able to treat the last part. This is where I was able to help him. I was able to treat the inflammation, residual pain, and the residual pocket of infection, increase the blood flow, and restore proper function in his groin area.

Western and Eastern medicine make such a great team. It is a shame that most medical professionals believe their own medicine has all of the answers. Due to this type of thinking, the only person who suffers is the patient. Working together to help patients is how it should be. This is how I approach all of my patients. My goal is to help them, not put ego first.

STIFF NECK

MAIN COMPLAINT

A 37-year-old man woke up with horrible neck pain. He had slept wrong. The pain is bilateral at C2-5, and on the lateral side of the neck on the cervical vertebrae. It hurts to flex, rotate, and extend his neck. He is having a hard time driving and turning his neck.

MERIDIAN INVOLVED /THEORY

Since this is an acute case, we only need to consider how to treat the BL, Du, and perhaps the KD. However, the KD channel is usually involved more with chronic pain issues. (Muscle tendino, channel relationships)

We need to treat C2-5, including the medial and posterior scalene muscles. Do not forget that the posterior scalene is controlled by the TW.

TREATMENT POINTS

Same side	77.01
	77.02
	77.03
	22.03
	So Jing Dian
Opposite hand	22.01
	22.02
	Ren 24

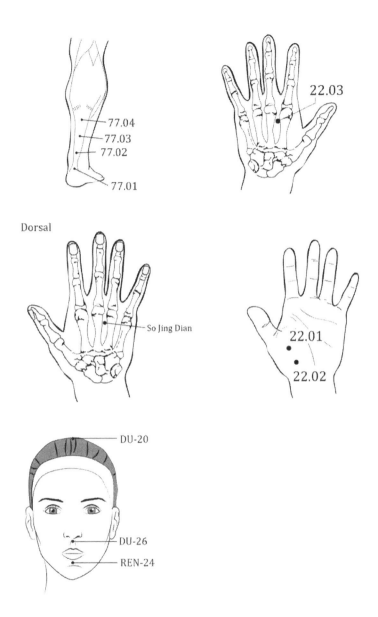

OUTCOME

He had a 95% reduction in pain while on the treatment table. He was able to turn his head, flex, and rotate his head with no pain. He still had pain when he extended his head backwards slightly, but he was happy that he could now turn his head without experiencing any pain. Since the treatment was on a Friday, I told him to call me next week if his pain comes back, but it should not return.

COMMENTS

This is the *only* time I ever see 22.01 and 22.02 work very well, when we are treating upper cervical issues. The wrist is the hand, so the palm of the hand is the upper neck. The LU channel treats the BL. These are very effective points for upper C1-7 pain, but not trapezius pain. You can use 11.09, instead of 22.01 and 22.02 for trapezius pain.

Points 77.01, 77.02, 77.03 are perfect for this type of neck pain. The BL channel treats the same side BL channel. We tap the bone to treat the bone pain. It is located in a huge tendon, the Achilles tendon, which resembles the neck tendons. These are fabulous points for neck pain. You could treat the opposite side as well, but I have found that the same side is more effective.

Ren 24 is important in this case. The Ren fixes Du, and the front treats the back.

Point 22.03 is indicated for neck pain, as is So Jing Dian. The knuckles of the hand where these points are located image the base of the neck, such as the GB 20 and BL 10 area.

Unfortunately, the term "fallen pillow syndrome," which 22.01 and 22.02 are indicated for, has been expanded into being used for typical trapezius pain. In my experience, these points will not effectively get the job done. Yes, there is a micro image of the palm being the upper back, and the channels work. You will hear or read that these points get trapezius pain, but it will be the exception and not the rule that your patients get adequate relief from these points for trapezius pain.

These points are also effective for shoulder pain. They do work well for that, in addition to neck pain. They even work well for scapula pain, but *not trapezius* pain, which so many people have.

TEMPORAL HEADACHE

MAIN COMPLAINT

My new patient does not know what she wants to treat. She is 55 years old and is dealing with left temporal headache radiating into her left trapezius muscles. I am too busy today to explain how and why acupuncture will help her. I have decided to let the needles speak for me. I have kept her in the chair, have her sign a quick waiver, and will treat her. I will leave her to treat my next patient, come back, and see how she feels.

She is currently in severe pain, a 7/10 on the pain scale. She is squinting her left eye because it hurts so much. She is also touching the left side of her head because it hurts. I have no idea why yet. I do not have the time to get to the root cause of her pain, but I need to prove this treatment works in order to get her to allow me to treat her further, so that I can determine the root of her problem.

POINTS USED

Opposite hand	22.03 22.04 So Jing Dian TW 3 SI 3 HT 7, HT 6, HT 5, HT 4 (needled from the SI channel into the heart channel)
Same side hand	San Cha San 11.16
Same side leg	77.05 77.06 77.07
Opposite leg	deep 66.03, 66.04 down to 55.02

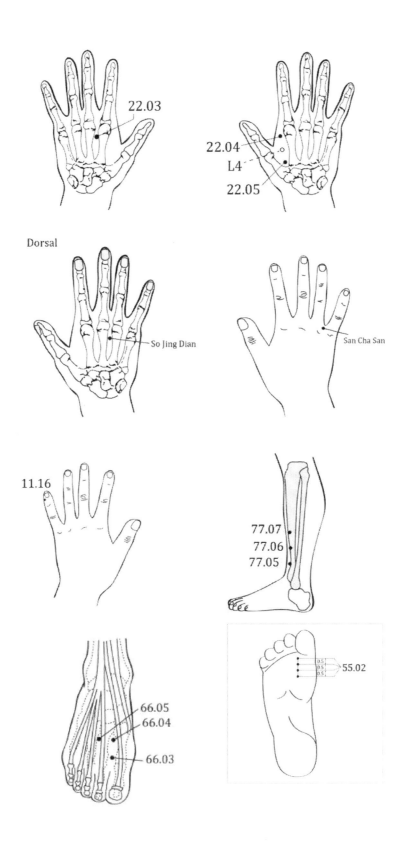

I let her sit with those needles for 5-8 minutes. When I returned to her, she is smiling and moving her upper neck and back. She is moving her head around, and she says that for the first time in weeks she does not feel her head.

I have rescheduled her for a longer appointment time to find out the root of her problem. I need to review her full medical history, and delve into what is happening to her medically.

This is a great case because sometimes you have to "put up or shut up." My patient did not care about anything. She was not listening to me, or paying attention because of her pain. She did not care about the root of the problem or the needle, or her Zang Fu issue. I do not even think she really wanted acupuncture. However, it is in cases like this when distal acupuncture and Tung acupuncture are mind blowing. She was astounded that I did not need to touch her head.

This is an example of how you can open yourself up to criticism. If the acupuncture works, that is great. She will be your patient for life. However, if the patient is like this and you fail, no matter what you say, she will never come back.

This is how I like to treat patients who do not believe what amazing medicine acupuncture is. I let the needles talk for me.

I assumed by palpation that most of the pain was coming from the base of her head, and arching over the head along the BL and GB meridians, into her temples and eyes. Points 22.03 and 22.04 are perfect, and they image the base of the head.

The point, So Jing Dian, as taught to me by Dr. Tan, is the image of the base of the head. TW 3, while not commonly used for this, also treats the base of the head, as does SI 3. All the knuckles get the base of the head. It is a perfect image.

Her pain also went into the trapezius muscles. The GB channel controls the trapezius muscles, using TCM theory. The BL channel controls the trapezius muscles via the muscle tendino channel theory.

Regardless of what theory you would like to use, needling from the SI to the HT, I can treat both channels. The SI channel gets the BL, and the HT gets the GB. The image is perfect. The lower arm images the upper neck. The SI channel will also treat the levator scapula which is controlled by the SI.

I used the same side San Cha San as a guide for the same side channel TW, which controls the posterior scalene. Point 11.16 is almost like SI 1. In Tung acupuncture, we use it for knee pain, heart issues, and stress. I liked it here for her stress component, and the fullness in SI channel (this will drain it). It is also a guide point for the SI pain in the upper neck.

The same side 77.05, 77.05, 77.07 is between the GB and ST channels. It is probably one of the few points in Tung system that is indicated for upper back pain. I like these points because they move all stagnation. They move all Qi stagnation, break masses, and treat the trapezius. I treat this point on the same side, because the pain is in the upper trapezius, which is controlled by the GB channel in TCM theory. The image of the lower leg images the upper back.

The points used on the opposite leg were a deep 66.03 and 66.04 going down to 55.02. She had eye pain, and 55.02 is indicated for eye issues. You can also needle from the top to activate 66.03 and 66.04, and then needle deeper to activate 55.02. I use this every day in my practice. Points 66.03 and 66.04 are much like LV 2 and LV 3. There are many different indications, but in this case, I used them for her blood and Qi stagnation, eye issues, stress, and face pain.

The patient will be back next week, at which time, we will start a regular course of treatment.

FOLLOW UP

This patient was very happy and surprised that her headaches, neck, and shoulder pain are much better. The pain is less sharp, her range of motion has improved, and she has not had a headache since I last saw her. Her trapezius muscles are good on the right side, but still tight on the left. She is still stunned that I have not put needles in her head or neck.

Today, she does not have a headache, but I decided to treat her as if she did. We can use points that will treat her trapezius pain, and also her headaches, even though she does not have one.

I did left side 77.26, the seven tigers, which are great for upper trapezius neck pain. The BL channel treats the BL, it is a three-point unit. All three points were used. The image of the lower leg is the image of the upper back.

Since the pain is on the BL channel, and we are using the BL channel to treat the pain, I chose points on the same side, this is known as System Six. The BL channel treats the BL. It will also treat the opposite side KD channel, which is still important because she used to hurt on both sides.

Left side	77.26 San Cha San
Opposite side, right	77.18 Tou points all 4 points

Hou Tou	Occipital headaches – fifth finger
Pian Tou	Temporal headache – fourth finger
Ding Tou	Vertex headache – third finger
Qian Tou	Frontal headache – index finger

73

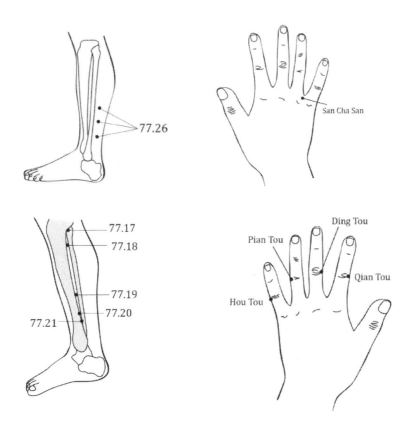

I used 77.18 on the opposite side, the right side. This is a great point for overall pain, inflammation, and arthritis. This will also help with her headaches, so that they do not come back. The SP treats the ST and TW channels. It is related to her kidney reaction area, and the kidney, via the five elements. All of these elements are important for this patient.

The four Tou points were used on the right hand, to cover her whole head. These four points are one point on each finger. They are great, mostly for headaches. Here I used them because I think most of her headaches, neck, and trapezius pain comes from her head.

We did San Cha San on the same side, as an opener, or guide. It is also a treatment point for the trapezius, posterior scalene, neck, and head.

After this treatment, she was 100% relaxed and out of pain. She could still feel the lump in her neck, but her shoulder and neck did not hurt. She will be back next week. I am going to treat her two more times over the next ten days. I will then re-evaluate her to determine if she needs further care.

GOUT

MAIN COMPLAINT

A 47-year-old man has gout. The gout is constant. Today it is affecting his big, right toe. His big toe is red, hot to the touch, and painful when touched.

MERIDIAN INVOLVED /THEORY

The SP and LV meridians in the big toe are the affected meridians. The cause of his gout is reduced kidney function. His kidneys are not able to break down uric acid.

POINT USED

Right side	88.09 88.10 88.11
Left side	77.18 77.19 77.21 11.27 points 1-2 (start counting these points at the distal end.

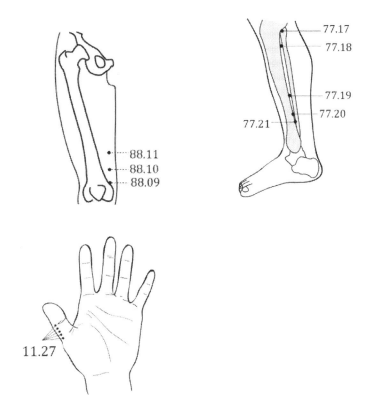

ADDITIONAL POINTS

The points were treated on each joint of the left thumb. Both the radial and ulnar side were used. I used six needles total, on the distal, medial, and distal joints. Another option for point selection would have been points 11.27 one to two. Both of these would be effective. These are not TCM or Tung points per se; I have modified them based solely on image and mirror concepts.

OUTCOME

I was able to relieve all his pain while he was on the treatment table. I took his pulse after the treatment, and his kidney pulse was better, and he had improved blood circulation. For a more lasting result, I would need a little

77

time. If he has a recurrence of the pain, I advised him to come back and I will do bleeding therapy locally, in his big toe.

COMMENTS

This is a great case. It demonstrates how we are treating pain, but the underlying cause is an internal disorder. His kidney function is declining, he has a poor diet, and is not able to get regular acupuncture treatments. As acupuncturists, we often have to deal with these types of things. We have to adjust our treatment plans for patients who cannot get regular care. Our patients also have dietary issues affecting the treatment outcome.

This patient was busy, he would only come for treatments in the morning, and he preferred to take herbs. He did not want to reduce his high intake of meat and beer. These factors continued to exacerbate, and perhaps even cause his gout.

The most important thing to focus on was kidney tonification. In Tung acupuncture, we apply the five-element theory of strengthening the kidney by supporting the spleen. You can see that points 88.09, 88.10, 88.11, and 77.18, 77.19, 77.21, are all on the spleen channel. The spleen channel treats the kidney channel.

Also, I did not use the same set of points, 88.09, 88.10, 88.11 bilaterally. In TCM, we treat the kidney on both sides. Your clinical success will skyrocket if you do not use the same Dao Ma bilaterally. Choose different Dao Mas, with different images, different reaction areas, with as much variety as possible. In this case, we used 88.09, 88.10, 88.11, and then a different set of points, 77.18, 77.19, 77.21.

Here is something else to consider. Do you think this patient cares that I treated his kidneys? No, he does not. Do you think he cares that we talked about why he has gout, how his diet affects it, his kidney function, poor blood flow, and weak kidney Qi? (Qi in this case refers to function). No, he does not. What does he care about? The pain in his big toe!

As practitioners, we know we need to treat his kidneys. However, as practitioners and human beings, we need to listen to our patients. His complaint is what we call the branch, not the root.

His only complaint was the pain in his big toe, the branch. By needling all thumb knuckles, his pain was immediately gone. Could I have used fewer needles on just 11.27, points one and two? Yes, I could have.

The patient needs to change his diet in order to prevent a possible recurrence. He also needs more treatments to tonify his kidneys and get his body functioning at a higher level. The thumb here treated the branch, which was his main complaint - his toe pain. The thumb is the best mirror for the big toe. As Dr. Tan says and I agree with him, when it comes to fingers and toes you can forget about channels, just mirror, it is that powerful.

Hip Pain in a 74-year-old

MAIN COMPLAINT

An 74-year-old woman fell in August. She had x-rays and MRIs, which revealed that nothing was broken. Her pain has come and gone since then. However, her pain level has increased dramatically since December. She has been in constant pain since then. She cannot sit, she can barely walk, and she also walks with a visible limp. Her pain is on the right side greater trochanter. There is possible bursitis, trauma, and inflammation of the head of the femur. Her bursa appears to be inflamed.

MERIDIAN INVOLVED /THEORY

GB, BL meridians from her fall SP meridian because of her dampness and inflammation on the left side

TREATMENT POINTS

This patient was older and very weak. She was not able to get up on the treatment table. I treated her in the chair, and was only able to treat her arm. She had pantyhose on her legs, and she was in too much pain to disrobe.

Opposite side (right shoulder)	LI 15, and one cun below SJ 14 and one cun below (TW) SJ 10 and one cun below
Opposite side right	Gu Ci Yi Gu Ci Er Gu Ci San San Cha Yi San Cha Er San Cha San 22.05 – Ling Gu

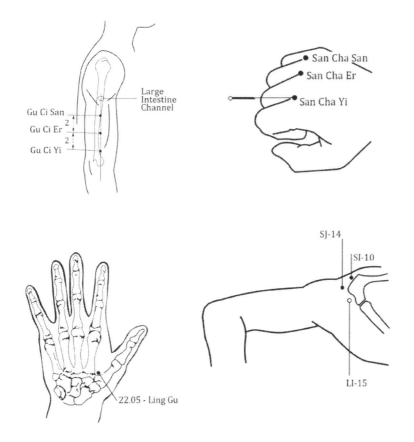

COMMENTS

This case was very interesting because patients usually experience an 80-100 percent pain relief during the treatment. Since this patient only had pain when she moved, she was not able to determine if her pain was gone while the needles were in. When we were done, she stood up and moved around. She said she felt better. By the time she got to the front door, all her pain had come back.

I felt as though the treatment did not work. I even told her, I am sorry, I have failed you, and I will need to treat you again. If you want to give up I understand, but I am the one who has failed you, not Chinese medicine. Please go find another practitioner. She understood and we decided to treat her one more time, three days later. (She was cash pay and did not have a lot of money.)

In most cases, if you provide treatment and the pain does not go away right then, it usually does not go away later. However, when I saw her three days later, she came to tell me she did not need the appointment. She said later on that evening she felt better and went to bed early. When she woke up, her pain was completely gone. It had not come back at all since the treatment, even though right after the treatment she had reported she did not really feel better.

I had the same experience with Tung acupuncture. An experienced distal teacher treated my bilateral KD 3 and KD 10 and bilateral HT 3 and HT 7. This is for bilateral low back pain caused by KD, BL, and GB meridian pain. During my treatment, I felt nothing. After the treatment, I still hurt. I figured it just did not work. That night I felt better, and the next day my pain was completely gone. I did not have back pain after that for the next three years.

What we can expect is that typically, the pain will instantly disappear. However, sometimes it does not. This is why I always suggest 2-3-4 treatments. After this, we are better equipped to determine progress.

The points chosen for the shoulder were based on the homologous image of the shoulder, which is just like the hip. To treat the shoulder, insert needles into the hip. The elbow, where Gu Ci Yi, Gu Ci Er, Gu Ci San are, is the image of the low back. This is also the reaction area of the Du, and tapping the bone will treat the bone, and the KI and GB channels. The points San Cha Yi, San Chi Er, San Cha San are the image of the low back. The wrist is the L5/S1 joint. The hand represents the hip and the low back. By needling all three San Cha points, I was able to treat all possible channels.

This is a great example of how we only have one or two chances to get results in our modern clinics. You need to make sure you get it. That is why I was redundant with my images. The shoulder, elbow, and the wrist all treat the hip. I was redundant on my channels. I used the LI, TW, SI, KD, GB and bone relationships.

I also treated more than just her hip, as she had requested. I assumed that she injured her hip when she fell. In addition to this, her low back and legs were affected. (San Cha San treats the lower leg pain). I treated her blood circulation (San Cha Er is the heart), as well as the Du channel, even though the Du channel does not treat the hip. We must listen to our patients, but not completely trust their perceptions.

The Gu Ci Yi, Gu Ci Er, Gu Ci San combination treats the KD, via the LI and KD. It is the reaction area of the Du/spine. The image is the low back and hip.

All San Cha points image the hip, treat the GB, BL, and KD channels. They also treat LU, HT, SP, and LV organs.

Ling Gu, 22.05, is the image of the low back. It is also the reaction area of the kidney, liver, ischium, lower jiao, and it is in one of the twelve segments.

All of these points not only treated the patient's branch, which is her hip pain, but also her root.

I have not seen this patient again. I do not think it was chance that her pain did not come back, or her body just needed that extra push. In my experience, for one in 70 patients, one treatment is enough to cure them. I do not know why, but no matter what it is, or why it is, or how long it is, the ratio seems to be 1/70. Whether I am treating back pain or Parkinson's, one of seventy patients will need just one treatment.

Knee Pain and Scheduled for Surgery

MAIN COMPLAINT

A 40-year-old female has bilateral knee pain, her left knee is much worse. It hurts all over, but she is scheduled for knee surgery in two months. Most of the pain is deep in her knee joint, in or around the patellar tendon.

She also has pain at the BL 40 area, the GB 34 area, and also proximal to the knee, at TCM extra point He Ding area. It hurts to walk, jump, and move. She is super fit, and appears to be strong and healthy. She does not take medications, and has no other diseases. She is very aware of her body, and cognizant of what makes her pain better or worse. She is very active and does martial arts, runs, hikes, goes snowshoeing, and works out regularly.

MERIDIAN INVOLVED /THEORY

ST, GB, BL and LV channels on the knee
Arthritis, degeneration, fluid, and edema of the leg
Overuse, and general degradation of the bone and joint

TREATMENT POINTS

Opposite elbow, shoulder, fingers and same side guide points, with anti-stress points.

First treatment:

Opposite side	44.06
	33.12
	LI 12, LI 11, LI 10
	11.09
	11.13

	22.08
	22.09
	Si Shen Cong
	Ear Shen Men
Same side	ST 43
	77.08

Treatment frequency: once per week

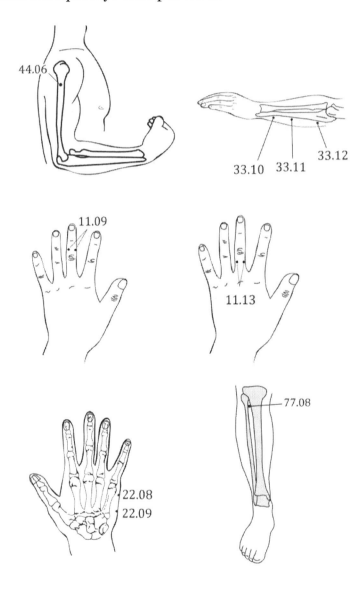

Second treatment:

Opposite side	PC 6
	PC 5
Same side	ST 43
	66.03
	66.04
	77.08
	77.09

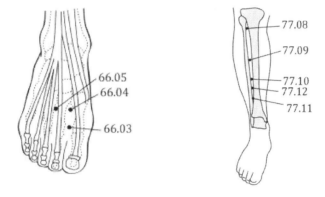

Third treatment:

Opposite side	Treatment points on the opposite leg, at the same location of the pain on the affected leg
Same side	88.25
	77.08
	77.09
	Si Shen Cong
	Ear Shen Men

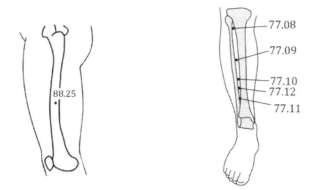

Treatments 4 and 7 were a repeat of first treatment
Treatments 5 and 8 were a repeat of the second treatment
Treatments 6 and 9 were a repeat of the third treatment

Treatment stopped after treatment 9, for her knee pain. She continues to come in. More on this later.

OUTCOME

This patient cancelled her knee surgery. I now treat her significant other, four of her friends, and she also comes in every two weeks just for stress. She also likes the good feeling she gets from acupuncture, the quiet time she gets lying on the table, and the general health benefits. Less stress, better sleep, increased energy, and better digestion are the four main side effects of all acupuncture, whether you are treating that or not. These things just happen. We also we keep the inflammation down on her knees so they do not start to hurt again.

COMMENTS

The knee can be imaged on the arm. Again, I used redundant and overlapping images. The lower leg can be imaged on the whole arm. This is a half image/half the leg, on the whole arm. The knee is right at the deltoid. It is on the LI channel, the LI channel treats the ST channel.

The elbow is a one for one image. The elbow is the knee. Since her pain was at the knee and above, I needled at the joint, and above and below it, LI 12,

LI 11, and LI 10. Point 33.12 is on the SI channel, the SI will treat the SP and BL, and the image is perfect.

I do not normally use TW 10. Why? Have you ever bitten your TW 10 area? You cannot feel anything. There are no nerves there! Acupuncture works by stimulating nerves, and if there are no nerves to be stimulated, it will not work well. I have never seen outstanding results with TW 10, so I no longer use it.

Points 11.09, 11.11, and 11.13 are on the PC channel. The PC treats the ST. From an image standpoint, it is hard to support the use of these points for knee pain. However, you have to remember that it is good to know why, but we also need to remember that it sometimes does not matter why. All that matters is that it works.

Points 22.08 and 22.09 are wonderful points for pain in the area of BL 40. The SI channel treats the BL. It is also the reaction area of the kidney.

I used Si Shen Cong and ear Shen Men because the patient was a bit stressed. I believe that it helps to relax patients. It is similar to how Gan Cao harmonizes in an herbal formula. It just makes the formula work better. The points Si Shen Cong and Ear Shen Men just make the treatment better, overall.

The guide point of 66.05 is the Shu stream point. It helps guide the pain to the knees. Did we use a local point? Points 77.08 or 77.09? It is right there, correct? It is basically ST 36. Is it OK? Yes, it is close to the knee pain, but not on the painful area. Therefore, it is OK. This is what we call a *close distal* point.

Not many Tung points are like this, but a few are somewhat *close distal* points. These points are so effective that you cannot *skip* them. Point 77.08 is great for knee arthritis. The point is close to the bone, thus it "cuts" the bone. It cuts bone spurs.

PC 7 and PC 6 increase circulation. It is a quarter image. It is the whole lower leg on one quarter of the arm. There is a big median nerve and tendon there, just like the patellar tendon. Like for like. The PC channel treats the ST channel.

Our same side points, 66.03 and 66.04, are on the liver channel. They are located right over the dorsalis pedis artery, which is a big vessel. They will increase blood circulation throughout the knee joint. The PC and LV talk to each other, and the LV will treat the knee itself, helping with tendons in general.

Another theory in Tung is to treat the same location of the pain, but on the opposite side. You would also add 88.25 on the same side as the pain. The brain will treat the opposite side of the body. Research backs up this ancient claim.

I think treating limb pain using this theory, is one of easiest and most reliable treatment principles. If I could, I would just open a clinic and treat only limb pain. It is almost 100% successful every time, with minimal treatment. In my experience, the best option of the Seven Channel Relationships is to treat limb pain with System One. This is also called Name Pairs. An example of this is the LU treats the SP, and the HT treats the KD.

System One
Chinese Meridian Name Sharing, from Dr. Richard Tan

Meridian	Meridian
Du	Ren
Heart	Kidney
Lungs	Spleen
Pericardium	Liver
San Jiao	Gall Bladder
Small Intestine	Bladder
Stomach	Large Intestine

The patient no longer has knee pain. She continues to exercise regularly and do all of the things that used to cause knee pain.

Treating points on both sides of the body does not cancel out the effects of distal acupuncture. If you treat one side and the pain is gone, ask if the pain on the other side is gone as well. If it is gone on both sides, you are done. If you still have pain, you can also treat the opposite side. This will not cancel out your distal treatment.

When I treat this patient, we are changing our image, relationships, treatments, and reaction areas. We *are* treating the whole knee even though the patient said it only hurt in an isolated area.

Although I typically like to treat pain patients twice a week, I only treated this patient once a week, and she did great. If I had treated her once a week and not been making significant progress, I would have asked her to come in twice a week, until we were able to get the pain under control.

Low Back and Rhomboid Pain in Pregnancy

MAIN COMPLAINT

This patient is 26 years old, and she is pregnant. I see her every two weeks. She has been my patient for several years. All previous health issues have been resolved. I have just been seeing her every two weeks to help treat any issue that comes up during her pregnancy.

Today, she has extreme pain in her right rhomboid and upper right neck. She also has pain in her lower back at her PSIS (posterior, superior, iliac spine) joints. Her lower back muscles, including the quadratus lumborum are also very painful. She is 34 weeks into her pregnancy. I believe this is the cause of her pain.

MERIDIAN INVOLVED /THEORY

Rhomboids-LI, SI, BL, KD and possibly the Du channel
Low back-Du, KD, BL, bone. The KD and bone being also GB

TREATMENT POINTS

Left side – opposite side	11.09
Same side	TW 3 and SI 3 (I don't like to do San Cha San on pregnant women it's just too much)
Bilateral	1010.19
	1010.20

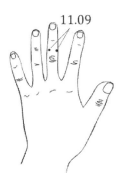 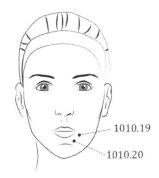

OUTCOME

First, the pain will come back, because she is pregnant. She walked into my office hunched over and limping, but walked out with no pain. Her back completely released with just 1010.19 and 1010.20 inserted bilaterally. Her pain will probably come back. My hope is that either it will not come back (maybe the baby will shift), or if it does come back, it will be less intense. Regardless, she was happy to be pain free.

Point 11.09 released the upper rhomboid pain. I prefer these points to 22.01 and 22.02. In my opinion, points 22.01 and 22.02 do not work very well, for upper trapezius, and rhomboid pain. They are more suited for upper cervical pain C1-7. I know many people think these points are effective and use them all of the time, but be careful. The only reason we should claim a point works, or does not work, is because that is what the patient reports to us. If the patient reports results, then I consider it a successful treatment. Just because some acupuncturists claim it works, or you read it in a book, does not mean it actually works. I do love 22.01 and 22.02 for asthma, fibroids, and yes, neck pain, but not T1-7 trapezius muscle, or rhomboid pain. It is much more effective for C1-7 pain.

It was quite remarkable how much pain this patient was in when she walked into my office. She was able to walk out of the office basically pain free. Her pain level was one or two on the VAS pain scale. It is also worth noting that this is where you will need to know the difference between theory and the practical application of acupuncture points. Sometimes the points you believe to be correct will not work like you expected.

93

Points 1010.19 and 1010.20 can be treated with one needle. You insert the needle from 1010.19 superficially to 1010.20. These points are primarily used for kidney issues and back pain. The image of the face can be broken down into numerous sections, and this section represents the lower jiao. The Pin Yin name also means to "water the kidney to pass through" (hence the indications for kidney issues). It is also the reaction of the kidney (the low back). These points image not only the lung, but also the kidney. This is why they also have the indications of asthma, breathing issues, kidney issues, and low back pain.

The middle finger is the torso of the body, and the posterior part of the middle finger is the spine of the back. The point 11.09 represents the upper back. Although a bit painful, it is remarkable for upper neck pain, and in particular, rhomboid pain. SI 3 and TW 3 were used as a guide. The treatment point was 11.09, and guides on the same side were SI 3 and TW 3. The pain was most likely on the SI and TW channels. Since the location of her back pain was the entire lower back, I used 1010.19 and 1010.20 bilaterally.

I will see the patient again in two weeks, and at that time, I will address any new concerns the pregnancy brings.

COMMENTS

It is interesting to note as to why her back hurt so much more during this second pregnancy, in comparison to the first one. Her last medical exam revealed that the umbilical cord was located too posterior, much more than normal. This was the cause of her severe back pain.

This is a good example of how acupuncture can be used as a diagnostic tool. Her back pain should have been resolved. Even for pregnant women, the pain will go away 90%, and stay away at least 50-90% of the pregnancy. In many cases, some of the pain will return, due to her pregnancy. This made me wonder what was really going on with her. Why was she not responding as she should?

Western tests show us, in this case, that we were doing acupuncture with the correct points. There must be something more serious, like a broken bone, cancer, a serious virus. In this case, the umbilical cord was very posterior, which is not normal. There was no way acupuncture needles would shift or move an umbilical cord.

This shows how when we do not get results, it is not because acupuncture does not work. It is not because it is TCM, Tan, or Tung that does not work. The problem is either the incorrect choice of points, or it is beyond something that we can treat. We should expect immediate, lasting, and effective results, all day and every day.

Neck Pain for Eight Years

MAIN COMPLAINT

A 47-year-old woman cannot move her upper neck. She is visibly stiff, and she cannot rotate her head. The pain is worse on the left side. She is wearing a neck brace to support and help her neck. She is visibly irritated, in pain, and not happy with life. She has had neck pain for the last eight years. She has been in constant pain, and her range of motion is restricted by 50%.

MERIDIAN INVOLVED /THEORY

Channel	Area It Treats
Du	Spine
KD	Deeper muscles of the neck
BL	More superficial neck muscles
SI	Levator scapula muscles
TW	Supraspinatus
SI	Infraspinatus
TW	Posterior scalene
BL and GB	Trapezius
BL	SCM, Sternocleidomastoid muscle
LI	Possible sub-scapular involvement
Jing Jin meridians	

There is blood stagnation, Qi stagnation, trauma, inflammation, dampness, swelling, stress, and tension. She also has degeneration of the bones, compression of the neck, and bone swelling.

TREATMENT POINTS

There are many issues with this patient. Her whole upper neck and back are affected. Even though she says it hurts on the left side, I know it is bilateral. We will just assume it is bilateral. My treatments for this patient are ongoing. We have been treating her for two months, twice a week. To date, she has had 16 treatments. Her pain is now 98% gone, with 100% ROM increased.

I wanted to highlight this case because I think this case would not have been as successful if I had only used 2-6 points for each treatment. I used a combination of Tan and Tung theory on her, which worked out great.

Same side	San Cha San
	22.03
	So Jing Dian
	SI 3
	-- I would alternate these points with Mu Guan/ Gu Guan and 11.11, depending on patient presentation.
	77.01
	77.02
	77.03
	77.05
	77.06
	77.07
	(I would alternate 77.05, 77.06, 77.07 with 77.26 and or 77.27, depending on the patient presentation of that day)
Same side, Opposite leg	SP 5, SP 5.5, SP 6
	LV 4, LV 5, LV 5.5, LV 6-- These points are perfect for typical American shoulder pain, I

	always use these.
Opposite arm	Alternate between HT 7, HT 6, HT 5, HT 4 and the set of points LU 10, LU 9, LU 8, LU 7, again depending on the presentation of the patient. I would add in or subtract 11.09 and 22.03
	Always treated Ren 24 and Du 24, Du 23, Du 22

This is a great case study, because it shows that with time and treatment, people will heal. This is also a great case study because the patient does regular lifting at her job, so she would re-injure herself every day. She injures her neck, upper shoulder, and upper back, on a daily basis. We would fix it and every day, she would re-injure it.

In a perfect world, where she did not continually re-injure her neck, one to three weeks with a few needles would have completely resolved her pain. However, with many patients working ten to twelve hours a day, five days a week, with no rest on the weekend, the body does not have a chance to heal.

I advised her that it would take longer to heal because she is repeatedly injuring the damaged tissue. We managed to take three steps forward and two steps back, long enough for her to stabilize and improve.

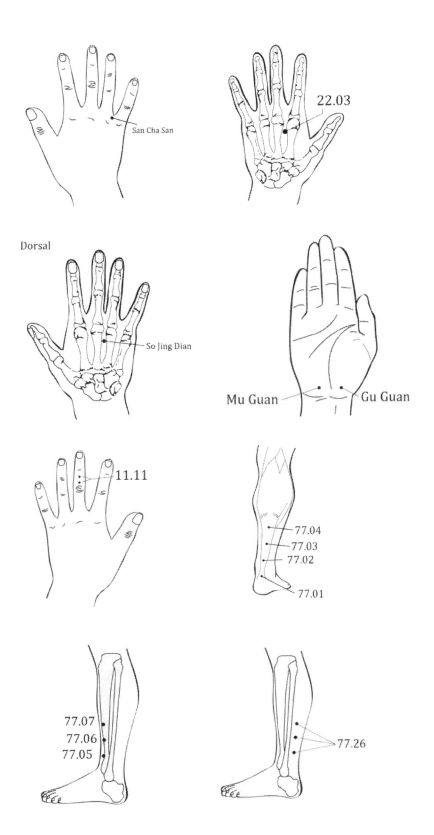

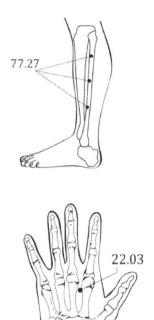

OUTCOME

She now comes in once a week, or every other week. She comes in to relax and remain pain free. She must continue her job, although she hates it, and it is too strenuous for her.

The root of her pain is a degeneration of the cervical bones. If they are left untreated, the pain radiates, and the muscles in her upper neck and back will hurt. As this pain progresses, she does not sleep, and she gets increasingly irritated, which just makes the whole situation worse.

Step one was get her to smile, which can get her out of pain. Step two was to reduce all her pain regardless of the root or branch. Step three was to address the root cause of her pain, and make sure it does not come back.

COMMENTS

Ren 24 treated the Du pain. The Ren will treat the Du. The front will treat the back. Du 24, Du 23, Du 22 also image the neck at C1-2-3-4. The Du meridian will treat the Du.

The same side hand points acted as my guide. San Cha San, 22.03, So Jing Dian, SI 3 all are guiding the same side channel, and the same side. This patient had bilateral head and neck pain, which is why we needed to treat both sides.

Mu Guan and Gu Guan are used for the boney arthritis swelling, and they also image the base of the neck. Points 77.01, 77.02, and 77.03 are my favorite neck pain points, especially neck pain in the C1-7 area. They treat boney, long-term, deep arthritic, and severe painful neck problems. These are on the BL channel, they treat the same side BL, and the opposite side KD. These points are so strong and effective that I think they treat everything in the neck. It is not channel directed. We tap the bone on this, so we are treating bone. They are amazing points.

Points 77.05, 77.06, and 77.07 are in between the GB and ST channels. Therefore, we will be able to treat both ST and GB indications, and channel relationships. The three weights are also for systemic pain, and systemic stagnation anywhere.

Dao Ma 77.27 is much like the three weights. It treats systemic stagnation and pain anywhere in the body.

Point 77.26 is on the BL channel, and is great for upper neck, upper trapezius, and upper sterno cleido mastoid pain. It is wonderful for upper neck pain. The image of the lower leg in this instance is the head. The foot is the head, and the ankle is the neck. The lower leg is the upper neck and upper back area.

These points are not Tung points. However, they are inspired by distal points, and follow Tung theory.

The TCM points SP 5, SP 5.5, and SP 6 treat the TW channel, the supraspinatus, and the posterior scalene. They also treat dampness. The SP has many other relationships as well such as the SI.

The LV channel is the main channel to use for the SI levator scapula, rhomboid channel, infraspinatus, and the SI channel. The image of the lower leg is the upper back. The LV treats the GB trapezius, and SI areas.

On the opposite arm, I would alternate between HT 7, HT 6, HT 5, HT 4, and the set of points LU 10, LU 9, LU 8, LU 7. This would depend on the presentation of the patient. I would also consider 11.09 or 11.11.

HT 7, HT 6, HT 5, HT 4 treat the GB channel, although you could also say that the GB channel runs through the neck. *When we treat pain, we are not treating the meridians, but instead, the muscle tendino channels.* The bladder channel controls the trapezius via the muscle tendino channels.

I still get great results by assuming that the HT channel will treat the GB. Remember, the wrist is C7/T1, so the area just proximal to the wrist represents the upper neck/upper back.

Last but not least, was the use of the LU channel. The LU is important because it treats the BL. It also treats the LI, which controls the rhomboids and subscapularis. The LI is not a channel we frequently think of when treating the upper back.

Did I use a lot of needles? Of course. I do not think that we can receive the best results with just treating a few things and hoping for the best. In modern clinics, most patients have multiple issues.

If we were able to treat a patient at the onset of illness, I think 77.01, 77.02, 77.03 and 22.03, along with 11.09, would have been enough. However, when a patient comes to you after eight years of neck pain, and you only have 2-3 visits to get them to believe in what you are doing, you need to get fast results. You need to view the treatment through the eyes of your patient.

What does your patient see? Does she see good results from your treatment? This is why we need a different approach with Tung needles.

FOLLOW UP

We have now shifted into a 12 magical treatment. This is a treatment taught by Dr. Tan, and it is great. I suggest you learn it. It is basically 12 needles, with one needle on each meridian, placed distal to proximal, and yin to yang. (See Dr. Tan's *book 12 magical*).

I like this treatment for this patient, because her pain is now gone. It is no longer in a specific area. We are just treating stress and some random aches and pains, as well as stiff joints here and there. By using the 12 magical, I can address her stress component and treat the entire body with just the 12 needles. It is working wonderfully. Her main issue was her left side neck pain.

Left side hand	HT 1
	PC 1
	LU 1
Right hand	LI 3
	22.03
	So Jing Dian
	San Cha San
Right leg	SP 5.5
	LV 5
	KD 7
Left Leg	BL 40
	GB 34
	ST 36

This is also a good example of how I use fewer and fewer points as patients heal. You can start with too many points, but we need to make sure that our patients heal as soon as possible.

But as they heal, muscles are healed and layers of pain are relieved. You can then reduce the number of points you use. I have many patients that had to have points treated on every limb. Now, we have one point on one limb, and one point combination on another limb.

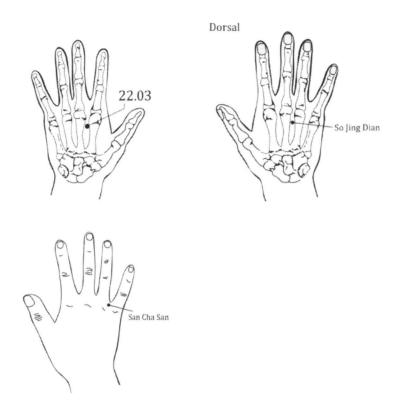

Today was an example of this. I had a long-term neck patient. All I need to treat now is 11.09 on the opposite side, with 77.26 on the same side. I have another back pain patient today who has been treated for two months. Her back is completely healed now. However, over time, as she ages, her pain might return. So I still treat her twice a month with opposite side 44.02 and 44.03, and same side 88.25. This is all that you need to treat as people heal. Remember to use as many needles as are needed, but as few as possible for an 85 to 100 percent positive outcome.

PLANTAR FASCIITIS PAIN AND STANDS ALL DAY

MAIN COMPLAINT

A 39-year-old man has bilateral heel pain located at the insertion point of the plantar fascia. Both heels hurt, but the left one is worse. He is a plumber who wears boots all day, and walks on hard surfaces.

He has had cortisone shots three times a year, for two years. The pain always goes away, but then it returns. He has taken pain drugs, but he does not like the side effects. It hurts when he walks all day. The pain is worse at the end of the day because he has been on his feet all day at work. The pain is worse at the insertion area of the plantar fascia, but it also hurts on the arch of the foot.

MERIDIAN INVOLVED /THEORY

The heel bone is the kidney. The Bone is KD, and possibly GB. However in this case, the KD pain is along the SP channel. Since it is tendon/fascia, we must consider possible LV involvement.

With any inflammation and irritation of the plantar fascia, it is important to be aware of a possible bone spur. We also need to think of the BL channel as well, even though most would say the heel is the kidney.

TREATMENT POINTS

Right side	Du 20, 3 needles at Du 20 and ashi points around Du 20
	Mu Guan, Gu Guan and 3 needles around the pisiform bone
	11.27 points 3-4-5. (Start counting from the most distal end)
Left side (pain side)	Same side insertion of SP 2 bilaterally for our guide LV 2 for our guide

Since the left side is worse, I started on the right side. The right side will treat the left side. It *might* also get both sides. We will treat the area, and then determine the results. He only hurts when standing. It will be hard to tell if we have resolved this problem, due to the fact that he is lying prone when the needles are in.

OUTCOME

The patient walked in, and as always, he enters with painful feet after a long day at work. After the treatment, he was able to walk out of the office with no pain. He was surprised at the lack of pain. Both sides were pain-free, even though we only treated one side.

He will come back three more times over the next 7-10 days in order to evaluate his treatment results and progress. Experience tells me that he will need 5-15 treatments for a 90% overall improvement. The high number of treatments is because this problem is so chronic. He is 80 pounds overweight, and he walks and stands all day on his job.

COMMENTS

This is an interesting case because it is a repetitive motion injury, which we can do nothing to prevent. He is a plumber, he has to wear boots, and he walks on hard surfaces all day. He needs to be pain free, and he cannot take the pain meds (because he hates the side effects, and legally he cannot perform his job on opiates). So, "Rocks are hard and water is wet." We need to fix him. Here we are, and we need to work with what we have. We have a tough situation.

Du 20 treats the heel because the head is the most yang. The foot is the most yin. Point 1010.01, or Du 20, is also an image of the heel. The top of the head gets the bottom of the foot. As we tap the skull at Du 20, we are tapping the bone at the heel. This will usually get both sides. Since the head does not decide which side to get, it gets both.

Mu guan and Gu Guan symbolize the foot. They are also for systemic bone swelling, arthritis, and systemic pain. It is bone for bone, and image for image. The head of the pisiform bone is actually the most correct homologous structure. This is why needling 2-3-4 Ashi points around the pisiform is extremely effective. In this case, the planter fascia was most sensitive at the anterior portion of the heel. When imaging on the hand, the pisiform bone is the heel. On the radial side of the pisiform bone, you will find the same image as the anterior part of the heel.

On the five-point unit, 11.27, of points 3-4-5, point 3 is just a "helper" and not really needed, but still, I always use it. Point 4 gets the foot and ankle. Point 5 is the heel. I like to use all three to make sure that I cover all of my bases.

A few notes on 11.27. It is a five-point unit. The Chinese name is Wu Hu, which means Five Tigers. Point 1 is the hand, point 2 is the wrist, 3 is really just a helper with no real indications, point 4 gets the foot, and point 5 gets the heel. That is why we reference 11.27 points 3, 4, and 5. It is the reaction area of the spleen, so it is very effective for damp, swelling, arthritic, and other painful conditions. These indications reflect the experience of these authors.

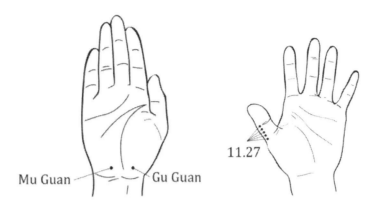

I chose SP 2 and LV 2 bilaterally as my guides to bring all the healing to the plantar fascia. My assumption was that the plantar fascia, though irritated, is not really the root of the problem, it is the branch. The root of the pain is the heel. If we can resolve the heel pain, then the arch pain should go away. I used the SP channel, because that is the channel of the foot arch. The LV channel was treated because that meridian could be involved in this pathology. The LV also treats the tendon and fascia.

Do not forget that yin points will get the same side, and the opposite side. Yang points only get the opposite side. I still do not like to rely on the yin points getting both sides. In this case, Mu Guan and Gu Guan are both yin points; I got lucky that they treated both feet.

Yin points treat *both* sides

Yang points treat only the *opposite* side

Regarding the choice of opposite or same side, a quick and fun trick with Dr. Tan's system of balance is that the even number points get both the same side and opposite side, and the odd numbers get only the opposite side. Dr. Tan teaches six systems of balance. Although this is not the same as Master Tung, many of the principles are the same.

Even number points=both sides

Odd number points=only the opposite side

It is also very important to tap the bone on all of these points. Tap the bone at Du 20 and the Ashi points. Tap the bone at Mu Guan and Gu Guan, and tap the bone at 11.27 points 3-4-5. This patient's pain was so focused on the heel, the root of it was his bone pain. This is why it was so important to touch all of his bones.

I also used three images, being redundant. I used the top of the head as the foot, the palm of the hand as the foot, and the thumb as the foot. Be redundant, overlap your images, enlarge your image, cover your bases, use multiple theories, and multiple treatment ideas. This is a long-term, chronic problem. It will be more complicated than the patient expects.

FOLLOW UP

At this time, this patient does not have any pain. He has returned to my office to work on his Hepatitis C. I was aware that he had this problem, but I knew that if I could not relieve his heel pain, he would not believe I could help him with something more complicated, such as Hepatitis C. This is an example of how treating pain successfully in your patients will gain their trust that you can treat other diseases.

I treated his heel pain six times. I think if we stop treatment, his pain will eventually return. The repetitive injury from his job, as well as his weight will continue to put pressure on his heels. Even though we are now focusing on Hepatitis C, I can still use a few points that will treat the heel, inflammation, dampness, repetitive motion injury, and treat the liver - all at the same time. That is the beauty of the Tung system.

Teeth and Jaw Pain for an Unknown Reason

MAIN COMPLAINT

A 62-year-old man has long-term pain in his jaw and teeth. The teeth pain is caused by chewing and biting. He had already been to the dentist to rule out cavities, and any other possible dental issues. He also had x-rays to rule out bone issues or broken teeth. His dentist thought it was from TMJ pain, and told him to follow up with his medical doctor. He came to see me before going to his medical doctor. His diagnosis was idiopathic teeth pain.

MERIDIAN INVOLVED/ THEORY

Areas of pain: upper and lower teeth, the back teeth more than the front teeth

ST meridian is the upper teeth
LI meridian is the lower teeth
Teeth are bone so you must treat kidneys
Bone is also related to gall bladder (per the Ling Shu)
You must needle bone to treat bone, because teeth are bone

Treatment principles: Focus first on the teeth. If the pain is not resolved, we will have to treat a possible TMJ issue, or some other problem.

POINTS USED

Opposite side	22.05 LI 4 22.04 (LI 3) 11.01, 11.02, 11.04 treat same side LI and gets opposite side ST 77.22 77.23
Same side	ST 45, ST 44 66.05 77.08 11.01, 11.02, 11.03, 11.04 22.05

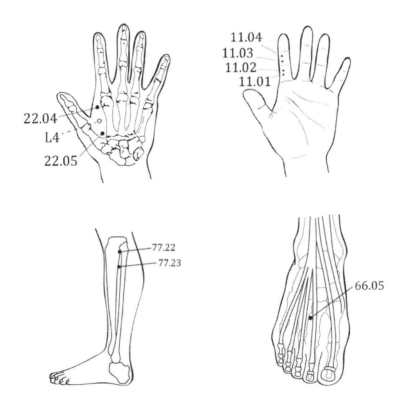

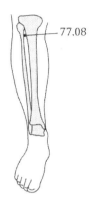

77.08

OUTCOME

This patient had 100% of the pain disappear while on the treatment table. I continued to treat him five more times. I treated him two times a week for two weeks, then once a week after the third week.

After this series of treatments, I told him that as long as his pain does not come back within ten days, it would not come back. We did not have to treat the TMJ aspect of his pain. I believe the root cause of his pain was the teeth.

I do not know the real cause of his pain. We both believe that it originated in an old root canal. He had a root canal three years ago. He had post-operative pain that would come and go. This time, it just did not leave. This is why he sought out treatment.

This case was interesting to me because there is a dental office next door to my office. I see a lot of teeth and jaw pain patients. It was wonderful to treat his LI channel (the hand is the face) and watch the same side lower teeth pain disappear, and the opposite teeth pain disappear.

When I inserted the ST points, I observed the same side upper teeth pain get better, and the opposite lower teeth pain get better. It is just fascinating to watch the process unfold.

The points 77.22 and 77.23 are perfect points for this. Since they are between channels, they get both the GB and ST. So even though we were not treating the GB related TMJ pain directly, we manage to treat it indirectly with these points. Points 77.22 and 77.23 are the reaction area of the teeth. The image in this instance is the whole face on the leg. The knee images the eyes. The points 77.22 and 77.23 are just below the knee, hence they are just below the eyes, and thus, they treat the teeth.

To pick up the kidney (bone), I used the LI channel. I did this because not only does the LI treat the LI, but it also the treats the ST. The LI also treats the kidney. In addition, when we treat 22.05, we insert the needle to the bone (tap the bone). By tapping the bone, we pick up the essence of the kidney/bone. The hand images the face, you can see that your first and second digits somewhat resemble the mouth of an alligator. By needling these points, we are treating the mouth.

This is a good case, because often we will not know the cause of the problem. We just need to treat, trust the points, and the body. We need to trust what the ancient doctors taught us, and hope for the best. We will not always know what the Western diagnosis is, but we can trust the body to heal itself with the right kind of help.

TRIGGER FINGERS FROM OFFICE WORK

MAIN COMPLAINT

A female patient, aged 45, has trigger fingers in the second and third fingers of her left hand.

MERIDIAN INVOLVED /THEORY

The channels involved are LI and PC. She has swelling of her fingers at her proximal and distal joints. The cause is unknown, other than wear and tear, or repetitive stress. Her husband is a banker and she works for him, so it is probable that her pain is caused by too much typing, filing, and other paperwork. Other than the trigger fingers, the rest of her health is relatively normal.

Today is her second treatment. During the first treatment, her fingers would click and stick as she flexed and extended them. After the first treatment, her fingers did not click or pop. She still had some soreness. She reported 20% remaining stiffness, but the clicking, popping, and sticking were gone.

She felt worse in the morning. Upon waking, her fingers would stick and pop. Throughout the day, her fingers would loosen up, but then progressively get worse, until eventually, at night her hand was inflamed and it was hard for her to grab things normally.

TREATMENT POINTS

First treatment

Same side	PC 9
	LI 11
Opposite leg	66.03
	66.04
	ST 44
	66.05
	66.06
	66.07

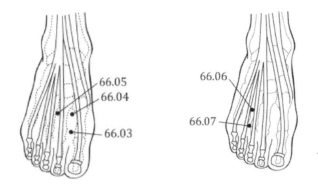

Second treatment

I wanted the patient to flex her fingers with the needles in, so I did not insert needles in the affected hand.

Same side leg	88.25
Opposite leg	66.03
	66.04
	ST 44
	66.05
	66.06
	66.07

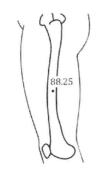

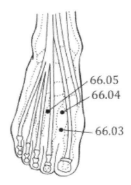

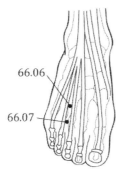

On the opposite leg, you could also forgo using Tung points, and just treat the exact spot on the toes that corresponds to the affected area on the hand. I prefer to use Tung points, but either way, I think would be just as effective.

OUTCOME

The patient will need more treatments. I would estimate, based on her results, that she will need two to four more treatments. It will take longer because she is older, not as active, and not physically fit. The patient had relief between treatments, as well as significant pain reduction.

COMMENTS

Points PC 9 and LI 11 on the same side "take out the fullness," and although not Tung points per say, they are Tung points in theory. They are applicable to the guiding needle technique.

Points 66.03 and 66.04 are like LV 2 and LV 3. They are similar, and they help treat the same points that are affected on the index fingers.

Points ST 44 and 66.05 treat the pain that is present on the hand at the web space of the second finger.

Points 66.06 and 66.07 treat the pain of the middle fingers.

For the second treatment, we kept the points the same, but added in 88.25 to help with systemic pain and inflammation. I could have used 11.27, and or PC 3, but I decided against using them. I like 11.27 for the reaction area of the spleen/damp systemic arthritic pain in hands and feet. PC 3 is usually great for thumb pain (As per Master Tung usage of TCM point PC 3), but it also works well for index and middle finger pain.

Today is the patient's third treatment. Her pain levels are reduced by 75% overall. She feels more pain in the third knuckle, in comparison to the rest of her hand. Her index finger is not an issue now. It does not make a snapping or popping noise, and it does not hurt. Her middle finger does not pop or snap any longer, but still there is some pain at the proximal metacarpal joint, on both sides of the knuckle.

For her third treatment today, we will mirror the third knuckle of the hand, on the third knuckle of the foot. I will also use 88.25 and 77.05, 77.06, 77.07 for systemic pain and stagnation. This is a great time, and if we wanted, to do reverse hand acupuncture.

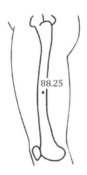

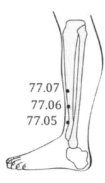

Think about this, the point So Jing Dian is right at the joint space of the third and fourth fingers. Luo Zhen, or 22.03, is right at the joint space of the second and third fingers. Both of these points, 22.03 and So Jing Dian, treat neck pain, do they not?

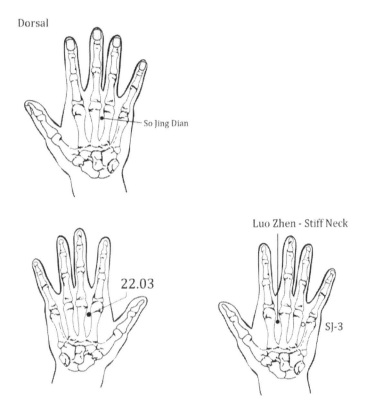

So we can theorize, and in practice it works, that if we needle the *neck*, we should be able to fix the proximal knuckle. If the knuckle treats the neck, why would the neck *not* treat the knuckle? Indeed, it works just great! If you needle GB 20 and BL 10 on the left side, it will fix the right proximal knuckle of the third finger. It is so interesting!

On the other hand, consider 22.08 and 22.09. These two points are used together, and are located between SI 3 and SI 4. These points treat many things, but one thing they are quite amazing for is popliteal fossa pain. OK, that makes sense. Therefore, if a person has pain at the SI 3 and SI 4 area, we would think that we could treat BL 65, BL 64, BL 63. However, we can also treat BL 40! BL 40 is the popliteal fossa, and doing "hand acupuncture in reverse" works great!

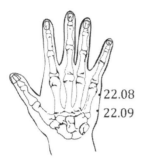

22.08
22.09

This will help you when your patient has finger or toe pain that is *so sensitive* you will not be able to needle the corresponding area. This is another example of why you need to know theory. If you just remember the points, you will be stuck. However, if you understand the theory of the points, you can work out a solution, such as working backwards. This gives you a lot more treatment options.

I often do "reverse hand acupuncture" when my patients have problems on their fingers and toes, and when they are not excited about having 5-10 needles in their extremities. We can just needle the corresponding area on the torso, in order to treat the area that the fingers or toes would have treated.

VARICOSE VEIN PAIN

MAIN COMPLAINT

A 37-year-old woman has pain in her blood vessels. She has varicose veins in her upper and lower legs.

MERIDIAN INVOLVED /THEORY

The liver and heart are the main organs to treat.

You could just find the meridians that run through the painful area and treat those, that would work, but to fix the root of this problem, you have to treat the weak blood flow in her heart. She also has a weak liver, and overall compromised blood circulation.

She has been coming to see me for stress and TMJ pain. Both of those issues have been resolved, and we are now focusing on her blood vessels, circulation issues, and the pain from her varicose veins.

OUTCOME

This is our seventh treatment for her blood vessel issues.

Right leg	88.12
	88.13
	88.14
	66.03
	66.04
Left leg	88.01, 88.02, 88.03 (every other treatment adding in 77.05, 77.06, 77.07)
Left arm	44.08,
	44.09
	44.10
Right arm	33.08 and 33.09 (every other treatment adding in 22.04 and 22.05)

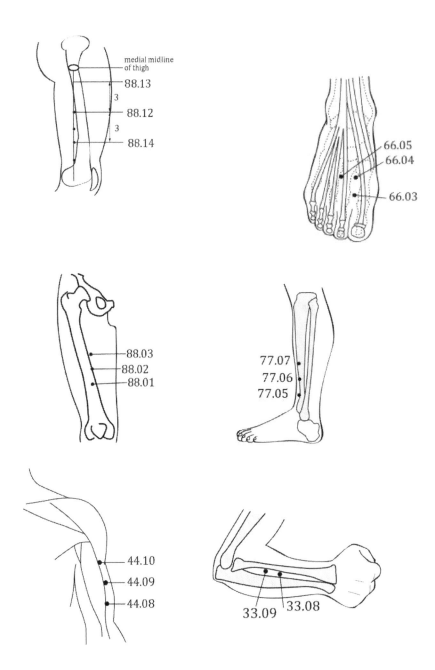

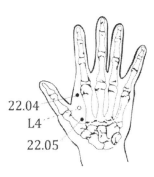

22.04
L4
22.05

The pain has been reduced by 75 % in her knees, thighs, and lower legs. Her veins are distended on different body parts, depending on what she has been doing, such as work, exercise, and sitting around. Usually her thighs, frontal and posterior knees, and lateral lower legs hurt.

I told her that I believed all her veins would be healthy in two to four more treatments. We may need to treat her once a month, for the next three to six months, depending on if she watches what she eats, exercises, and lowers her salt and fat intake, in addition to other lifestyle issues. The issue with varicose veins is that as long as the perforator valves are not broken, you can fix the distended vein. If the valve is broken, no matter how much you treat them, after 24 hours, the distention will come back.

I will continue with these points because I do not see the need to change them. I will only change them if the patient starts to complain about one particular spot that does not get any better. I will then have to reevaluate and refocus the treatment points.

COMMENTS

In many cases, I try to get the patients healthy enough so they can heal on their own. We have to remember why acupuncture and herbs were invented. It was said in the classics "they invented acupuncture and herbs" because "wine and prayer" were not enough." They needed a new way to "wipe away the dust" as they said; and that new way was "acupuncture and herbs."

Acupuncture and herbs were never meant to be used forever. They were meant to get you healthy enough so that you could get to "prayer and wine" in order to heal yourself. (Wine here is mentioned because of the vaso dilation and increased blood flow effect, not because drinking is a good thing. It is not. But minimal amounts of a vaso dilation effect is important for overall health. This means one glass of wine, per night, versus what some people do, which is five glasses of 12 ounce glasses of wine.

So the goal was to get her healthy enough to be able to exercise, move, be happy, eat better, and then, certainly the last 10 to 20% will be healed. If she exercises and eats correctly, she will not need treatment again. We just need to get her healthy enough, and get her out of pain, so that she can move.

The points are a good representation of a vessel for vessel. She has a vascular problem. The two organs responsible for this are the heart and liver. Points 88.01, 88.02, 88.03 treat the heart, ST for ST, the reaction area of the heart, and the image of the heart. There is the huge femoral artery here at these points.

Points 88.12, 88.13, 88.14 are the reaction area of the liver, LV for LV, and the image of the LV. Of course, we treated 88.12, 88.13, 88.14, but on which side? The right side! Where is the liver? It is on the right side; LV for LV; same channel, same side. So, where then did I treat 88.01, 88.02, 88.03? What side is the heart on? It is on the left! ST channel for same side channel, ST for ST.

Consider points 66.03 and 66.04, 88.01, 88.02, 88.03, 44.08, 44.09, 44.10. Why are these points so amazing? They are all over large vessels. These include the dorsalis pedis artery, the femoral artery, as well as the brachial artery. If we want to fix a vessel issue, we need to treat around the vessels. These points are all indicated for increased blood volume, and increased blood flow.

We have mentioned many times using 22.04 and 22.05 for increased Yang qi, blood, and movement. Points 77.05, 77.06, 77.07, the three weights, break stagnation, and move Qi and blood. There is research that shows using

77.05, 77.06, 77.07 will increase blood flow to the head. It is interesting that one of the indications is for stroke and hemiplegia.

The reaction area of 44.10 is the reaction area of the legs, where her pain was. This is a very effective treatment. In addition, it is over the brachial artery.

Every time we did a treatment, her joint pain would be relieved. She would come in with heaviness, pain, and stiffness, but leave feeling pain-free. Even general aches and pains can be resolved within a matter of seconds. Many people believe that only a small spot of pain can be fixed instantly. Here we had multiple areas, multiple joints, limbs, and tissues. After about 50% of the needles were inserted, the patient felt warm, relaxed, and pain-free. This never ceases to amaze me.

Treating the problem, which is where she hurts, but also focusing on the root cause, will give you the most effective Tung treatments.

The person who says it cannot be done should not interrupt the person who is doing it.

–Chinese Proverb

CHAPTER THREE

HOW TUNG POINTS TREAT THE ROOT

Many distal theories and or strategies use the concept of balancing the channels, using the right image, and applying the correct theory to achieve the best results. You might ask if this addresses all aspects of the disease. The pain relief is easy to see. However, have we also treated the other diseases the patient might have? In Chinese medicine, we always treat the root. It is important to address other health issues that might be affecting the health of our patients.

There are over 300 points for back pain, and they all work. Which points would you choose if the cause of the pain were a spinal compression? Your first thought would be the Du channel. For this, we would use the points Gu Ci Yi, Gu Ci Er, and Gu Ci San. These points are the best choice, because the reaction area is the Du channel. It treats from multiple perspectives. It treats the low back from an image of the back, and arm.

They also treat from a channel perspective. The TW channel treats the KD. The TW treats the GB. However, they also treat the root. The root of the problem is the spine. The reaction area of these points is the Du channel, which treats pain on all levels, the branch and the root.

What would you do if the back pain is coming from a kidney deficiency? Would you be able to just pick images and channels in the back? In this case, we could choose points that treat the KD, BL, and GB channels, that go through the kidneys. Would that be enough to completely resolve the problem?

The best option is to do as Master Tung suggested, choose points that treat the kidney via the channel and image, but also that treat the kidney organ. Points 22.08 and 22.09 would be good points. These two points are on the SI channel, around the SI 3-4 area. This is the correct image, the lower hand treats the lower back. It is the correct channel. The SI channel treats the KD and BL channels. It treats the root, which is the kidney. Points 22.08 and 22.09 are the reaction area of the kidneys.

Reaction Area

The reaction area is very important in Tung acupuncture. This is the definition:

> "Reaction area" neuro-physical acupuncture. This reflects the knowledge of the delicate energy of the body and the neuroanatomical and neurophysiologic aspects of the body. This acupuncture style also corrects and heals the body through the manipulation of the peripheral and central nervous system by affecting the neuraxis, the actual anatomy, physiology and pathophysiology of the body. (Maher, *Advanced Tung Style Acupuncture*)

Ling Gu, 22.05, is a good example of this. The channel is correct. The LI treats the KD channel. The KD channel runs through the low back. The image is correct. The lower hand treats the lower back. The twelve segments and three jiaos all line up. Ling Gu is in the twelfth segment and the lower jiao, all where the low back is.

The question is, are you treating the root cause of low back pain? Yes. The reaction area is the ischium, and the lung. This also explains why Ling Gu is helpful for breathing, and blood circulation. Ling Gu, 22.05, is said to help yang Qi. It helps yang Qi because it is the reaction area of the lung. We can use this point to increase lung function (yang), and also increase blood and oxygen from the lungs to the heart and the rest of the body. When you increase blood, oxygen, and yang Qi, you are treating the root, the reaction area.

Brain Issues

For treating brain issues, there are many ways to image the head. Master Tung acupuncture has multiple images and channels that treat the brain.

There are also points that treat the brain, they include 66.13, 66.14, 77.01, 77.02, 1010.01, 1010.05, 1010.06, 1010.08. These points all treat the actual anatomy, physiology, and pathophysiology of the brain.

Diaphragm Issues

If you want to treat the diaphragm, you could just draw a line from the area where it intersects on the arm, and just insert a bunch of needles haphazardly in that area and hope for the best. We would also look at all the channels that run through the diaphragm and balance all of them. We could also treat the actual diaphragm, the body part. We would do this with 44.08, 44.09, 44.10. Point 44.10 is the reaction area of the diaphragm. It is a way to treat your patients on a much deeper level.

Fertility

There are two very famous points for fertility, points 11.06 and 11.24. The channels and images are both perfect. However, point 11.24 is the reaction area of the uterus, and 11.06 is the reaction area of the liver and kidney. That means these two points will treat three roots, the liver, kidney, and uterus.

Most of my patients who have infertility issues also have liver, kidney, and uterus issues. We can start to see why and how these Tung points are so powerful. The Tung system is so much more than just drawing a line, transferring an image, or just balancing a channel. These theories all work, but your treatments will vastly improve once you take it to the next level by looking at the root, and the reaction area associated with the disease.

The examples are endless. Do not ever think that Tung acupuncture just treats pain. The reaction area helps you decide which points to use. Check your channel, images, theory, and root cause of the disease. Once you have determined the root cause, you can choose the reaction area points. This will also ensure that the back pain that goes away on the treatment table does not come back. You will have treated the channels, but also treated the underlying patterns, which will heal the root cause.

Men have become the tools of their tools.

Henry David Thoreau

CHAPTER FOUR

TUNG POINT NUMBERING SYSTEM

People sometimes question the unusual numbering system of Tung acupuncture. If you think about it, the Tung system is no different from the TCM numbering system. If you compare the Tung point numbers to the TCM numbers of LU 7, SP 6, or St 36, you can see that it is only a matter of making sense of the system. You spent a year learning TCM points. You had teachers and other students to help you. You usually have to learn Tung points on your own, so it can be challenging.

The Tung numbering system, although it may seem odd, is not as strange as we think. It is helpful to learn the Pin Yin names. They communicate a lot of information about the points. An example of this is 11.07, 33.08 and 33.09, 66.05, 77.24 and 77.25. They all have a common indication. You cannot tell by looking just at the numbers, but if you knew Pin Yin, you would notice that they all have the word Jin in them. Jin, in this case, means digestion. All of these points treat digestive issues.

You are probably familiar with Zu San Li. It means three-leg mile point. The name ST 36 means nothing. However, if you know the meaning of the point name, you can infer that if you needle ST 36, you will have more energy and be able to walk more. Knowing the Pin Yin names of the acupuncture points, whether they are Tung or TCM points, can be very helpful to understand the functions.

Master Tung named points in two ways. Most of his points have a number and a Pin Yin name. About 25% of his points do not have a number. They only have a Pin Yin name. I do not know why. There are many theories as to why some of the points do not have numbers, but no one is sure.

The numbered points on the chest and back are not needled, ever. They are only used for bloodletting. You will see points on the chest and back using the initials DT or VT. DT is dorsal trunk, and VT is ventral trunk. Other authors devised these numbering systems so they would be able to use numbers, and avoid the necessity of using the Chinese names. Each author can use his/her own numbering system.

The numbering system on the body is as follows:

The fingers are 11.00.
The hands are 22.00
The lower arms (wrist to elbow) are 33.00
The upper arms (elbow to shoulder) are 44.00

The bottom of the foot is 55.00
The top and side of the foot is 66.00
The lower leg, from ankle to knee is 77.00
The upper leg, from knee to hip is 88.00
The ear is 99.00
The head and face is 1010.00

That is it! Therefore, if I were to say that I needled Men Jin, and knew Pin Yin, you would know what it does and where it is located. If you do not know Pin Yin, and I said I needled 66.05, you still do not know what it does. However, you could look it up. However, you will know that it must be on the top or side of the foot. It is in the 66.00 part of the body. The number 66.05 tells you that it is the fifth point listed for the foot. Easy!

There are other numbering systems out there. The numbering system I use in my clinic and in my books is the one taught to me by Dr. Wei Chieh Young. Dr. Young was a student of Master Tung. This numbering system is the one that is most commonly used. However, you will find there are other authors, disciples, students, and masters who use different numbers, different locations, and even at times some different names.

Some people use the name Master *Tong*, not Master *Tung*. There is even disagreement on his name! Remember that the important thing is that the effectiveness of the points is proven in clinic. If what you are doing is working, you can keep doing it. If it is not working, you should analyze, study, learn, open your mind, and expand your knowledge.

Sometimes I mention a different numbering system, such as a Dao Ma of the points BL 65, BL 62, BL 60 by Dr. Maher. That is a different numbering system. Another example of this is the Dao Ma by Dr. Maher, 88.01. That Dao Ma is the points 88.09, 88.10, 88.11, as noted by Dr. Wei Chieh Young. This is not to confuse you. It is just to bring attention to the numbering systems.

Dr. Maher numbered his Dao Mas in the same way that the points themselves are numbered. To differentiate the point numbers from the Dao Mao numbering from Dr. Maher, I will notate that it is a Dao Ma number.

You will see references to points that were used that were between regular acupuncture points. SP 5.5 is halfway between SP 5 and SP 6. LV 5.5 is halfway between LV 5 and LV 6.

Opportunity is missed by most people because it is dressed in overalls and looks like work.

Thomas A. Edison

CHAPTER FIVE

REACTION AREAS

These points were compiled from numerous resources, including some from the books by Dr. Wei Chieh Young, Dr. James Maher, and Dr. Henry McCann. We recommend you continue your studies to learn more about the reaction areas in these books.

A quote from Dr. James Maher:

"Reaction areas treat disorders of the organ in question (i.e. both the TCM and Western biomedical organ)"

And

"There are differing opinions amongst various Taiwanese and Master Tung experts concerning the reaction/nerve area of many of the points. Disagreement among the various authors is not uncommon and may merely reflect the evolution of Master Tung's research and teachings to his apprentices."

1010.01	Brain
1010.05	Brain
	Spine
	Cerebral
1010.06	Brain
	Spine
1010.08	Brain
	Facial motor nerve
	Heart
1010.09	Eyes
	Lungs
1010.11	Eyes
	Lungs

1010.11	Eyes Lungs
1010.13	Kidneys Lungs Bladder
1010.14	Kidneys Bladder
1010.16	Endocrine glands
1010.19	Spleen Kidneys *some texts also say Stomach and Liver
1010.20	Spleen Kidneys *some texts also say Stomach and Liver
1010.21	Heart Liver
1010.22	Lungs Kidneys Spleen
1010.25	Kidneys Liver
11.01	Heart Small Intestine Large intestine
11.02	Lungs Heart Six Fu
11.03	Heart Six Fu
11.04	Heart Six Fu
11.05	Lungs Heart Six Fu
11.06	Liver Kidneys

11.07	Lungs
11.08	Lungs
	Kidneys
11.09	Heart
11.11	Heart
	Lungs
11.12	Eyes
	Kidneys
11.13	Gall Bladder
	Heart
11.16	Gall Bladder
	Heart
11.24	Uterus
11.27	Spleen
22.01	Lungs
	Heart
22.02	Heart
	Lungs
22.03	Heart
	Lungs
	Liver
22.04	Lungs
22.05	Ischium
	Lungs
	*some texts show also the intestines and Heart
22.06	Kidneys
	Heart
	Spleen
	*some texts show as Liver and Bladder in addition
22.07	Kidneys
	Heart
	Spleen
	Liver
22.08	Kidneys
	Liver
22.09	Kidneys

	Liver
22.11	Kidneys
	Spleen
	Liver
33.01	Lungs
33.02	Lungs
33.03	Lungs
33.04	Heart
	Lungs
33.08	Lungs
	Liver
33.09	Lungs
	Liver
33.10	Liver
	Kidneys
33.11	Liver
33.12	Heart
33.16	Heart
	Lungs
44.02	Liver
	Heart
	Spine/Du
44.03	Liver
	Heart
	Spine/Du
44.06	Heart
44.08	Heart
	Liver
	Lungs
44.09	Heart
44.10	Legs-lower calf
	Six Fu bowels
	Diaphragm/flanks
44.11	Lungs
	Six Fu bowels
44.12	Kidneys

	Lungs
66.01	Heart
66.02	Heart
66.03	Heart
	Liver
66.04	Heart
	Liver
66.05	Stomach
	Uterus
	Duodenum
66.06	Spleen
	Liver
66.07	Spleen
	Liver
66.08	Lungs
	Kidneys
	Gall Bladder
	Liver
66.09	Lungs
	Kidneys
	Liver
66.10	Heart
	Kidneys
	Liver
66.11	Heart
	Kidneys
	Liver
66.12	Heart
	Kidneys
	Six Fu bowels
	Uterus
66.13	Heart
	Kidneys
	Six Fu bowels
	Uterus
66.14	Kidneys

	Brain
66.15	Kidneys
	Brain
77.01	Brain
	Spine
77.02	Brain
	Spine
77.03	Brain
	Spine
	Lungs
77.04	Heart
	Lungs
	Gastrocnemius
77.05	Heart
	Lungs
	Spleen
77.06	Heart
	Lungs
	Spleen
77.07	Heart
	Lungs
	Spleen
77.08	Lungs
	Heart
77.09	Heart
	Lungs
	6 bowels
77.10	Heart
	Lungs
	6 bowels
77.18	Kidneys
	6 bowels
	Heart
77.19	Kidneys
	Liver
77.20	Heart

	Kidneys 4 extremities Liver
77.21	Kidneys Liver
77.22	Teeth Lungs
77.23	Teeth Lungs
77.24	Larynx Pharynx Throat Thyroid Lungs Kidneys
77.25	Larynx Pharynx Throat Thyroid Lungs Kidneys
77.26	Thoracic cage Chest Ribs
77.27	Lungs
77.28	Kidneys Liver
88.01	Heart
88.02	Heart Stomach
88.03	Heart
88.09	Kidneys Liver
88.10	Kidneys Liver
88.11	Kidneys

	Liver
88.12	Kidneys
	Liver
	Heart
88.13	Kidneys
	Liver
	Heart
88.14	Kidneys
	Liver
	Heart
88.17	Liver
	Lungs
88.18	Liver
	Lungs
88.19	Liver
	Lungs
88.20	Lungs
	Facial motor nerves
88.21	Lungs
	Facial motor nerves
88.22	Lungs
	Facial motor nerves
88.25	Lungs
	4 limbs
88.27	Upper legs (both thighs and quads)
88.32	Throat
Ding Tou	Vertex
Fan Hou Jue	Lungs
Gu Ci Er	Liver
	Kidneys
Gu Ci San	Liver
Gu Ci Yi	Liver
	Kidneys
Gu Guan	Kidneys
	Lungs
Hou Tou	Occiput

Mu Guan	Kidneys
	Lungs
Pian Tou	Parietal and temporal
Qian Tou	Frontal head
San Cha Er	Heart
San Cha San	Spleen
	Kidneys
	Trigeminal nerve
San Cha Yi	Lungs

Chapter six

Tung Points list

(Bolded numbers are the most commonly used points.)

Number	Pin Yin
11.01	**Da Jian**
11.02	**Xiao Jian**
11.03	**Fu Jian**
11.04	**Wai Jian**
11.05	Zhong Jian
11.06	Huan Chao
11.07	Zhi Si Ma
11.08	Zhi Wu Jin
11.09	**Xin Xi**
11.10	**Mu Huo**
11.11	**Fei Xin**
11.12	**Er Jiao Ming**
11.13	**Dan**
11.14	Zhi San Zhong
11.15	Zhi Shen
11.16	Huo Xi
11.17	**Mu**
11.18	Pi Zhong
11.19	**Xin Chang**
11.20	Mu Yan
11.21	San Yan
11.22	Fu Yuan

11.23	Yan Huang
11.24	**Fu Ke**
11.25	Zhi Yan
11.26	Zhi Wu
11.27	**Wu Hu**
22.01	**Chong Zi**
22.02	**Chong Xian**
22.03	**Shang Bai**
22.04	**Da Bai**
22.05	**Ling Gu**
22.06	**Zhong Bai**
22.07	**Xia Bai**
22.08	**Wan Shun Yi**
22.09	**Wan Shun Er**
22.10	Shou Jie
22.11	Tu Shui
33.01	**Qi Men**
33.02	**Qi Jiao**
33.03	**Qi Zheng**
33.04	Huo Chuan
33.05	Huo Ling
33.06	Huo Shan
33.07	Huo Fu Hai
33.08	**Shou Wu Jin**
33.09	**Shou Qian Jin**
33.10	**Chang Men**
33.11	**Gan Men**
33.12	**Xin Men**
33.13	**Ren Shi**
33.14	**Di Shi**
33.15	Tian Shi
33.16	Qu Ling
44.01	Fen Jin
44.02	**Hou Zhui**
44.03	**Shou Ying**

44.04	**Fu Ding**
44.05	Hou Zhi
44.06	**Jian Zhong**
44.07	Bei Mian
44.08	**Ren Zong**
44.09	**Di Zong**
44.10	**Tian Zong**
44.11	**Yun Bai**
44.12	**Li Bai**
44.13	Zhi Tong
44.14	Luo Tong
44.15	Xia Qu
44.16	Shang Zu
44.17	Shui Yu
55.01	Huo Bao
55.02	Hua Gu Yi
55.03	Hua Gu Er
55.04	Hua Gu San
55.05	Hua Gu Si
55.06	Shang Liu
66.01	Hai Bao
66.02	Mu Fu
66.03	**Huo Ying**
66.04	**Huo Zhu**
66.05	**Men Jin**
66.06	**Mu Liu**
66.07	**Mu Dou**
66.08	**Liu Wan**
66.09	**Shui Qu**
66.10	**Huo Lian**
66.11	**Huo Ju**
66.12	**Huo San**
66.13	Shui Jing
66.14	Shui Shang
66.15	Shui Xian

77.01	**Zheng Jin**
77.02	**Zheng Zong**
77.03	**Zheng Shi**
77.04	**Bo Qiu**
77.05	**Yi Zhong**
77.06	**Er Zhong**
77.07	**San Zhong**
77.08	**Si Hua Shang**
77.09	**Si Hua Zhong**
77.10	**Si Hua Fu**
77.11	**Si Hua Xia**
77.12	Fu Chang
77.13	Si Hua Li
77.14	Si Hua Wai
77.15	Shang Chun
77.16	Xia Chun
77.17	Tian Huang
77.18	**Shen Guan = Tian Huang Fu**
77.19	**Di Huang**
77.20	**Si Zhi**
77.21	**Ren Huang**
77.22	**Ce San Li**
77.23	**Ce Xia San Li**
77.24	**Zu Qian Jin**
77.25	**Zu Wu Jin**
77.26	**Qi Hu**
77.27	**Wai San Guan**
77.28	Guang Ming
88.01	**Tong Guan**
88.02	**Tong Shan**
88.03	**Tong Tian**
88.04	Jie Mei Yi
88.05	Jie Mei Er
88.06	Jie Mei San

88.07	Gan Mao Yi
88.08	Gan Mao Er
88.09	**Tong Shen**
88.10	**Tong Wei**
88.11	**Tong Bei**
88.12	**Ming Huang**
88.13	**Tian Huang**
88.14	**Qi Huang**
88.15	Huo Zhi
88.16	Huo Quan
88.17	**Si Ma Zhong**
88.18	**Si Ma Shang**
88.19	**Si Ma Xia**
88.20	Xia Quan
88.21	Zhong Quan
88.22	Shang Quan
88.23	Jin Qian Xia
88.24	Jin Qian Shang
88.25	**Zhong Jiu Li**
88.26	Shang Jiu Li
88.27	Xia Jiu Li
88.28	Jie Xue
88.29	Nei Tong Guan
88.30	Nei Tong Shan
88.31	Nei Tong Tian
88.32	Shi Yin
99.01	Er Huan
99.02	Mu Er
99.03	Huo Er
99.04	Tu Er
99.05	Jin Er
99.06	Shui Er
99.07	Er Bei
99.08	Er San
1010.01	**Sheng Hui**

1010.02	Zhou Yuan
1010.03	Zhou Kun
1010.04	Zhou Lun
1010.05	**Qian Hui**
1010.06	**Hou Hui**
1010.07	Zong Shu
1010.08	**Zhen Jing**
1010.09	Shang Li
1010.10	Si Fu Er
1010.11	Si Fu Yi
1010.12	Zheng Ben
1010.13	Ma Jin Shui
1010.14	Ma Kuai Shui
1010.15	Fu Kuai
1010.16	Liu Kuai
1010.17	Qi Kuai
1010.18	Mu Zhi
1010.19	**Shui Tong**
1010.20	**Shui Jin**
1010.21	**Yu Huo**
1010.22	**Bi Yi**
1010.23	Zhou Huo
1010.24	Zhou Jin
1010.25	**Zhou Shui**

TUNG POINTS WITH NO NUMBER

Pin Yin
Ci Bai
Ding Ke
Ding Tou
Fan Hou Jue
Fei Qi Er
Fei Qi Yi
Fen Zhi Shang
Fen Zhi Xia
Fu Ge San
Gu Ci Er
Gu Ci San
Gu Ci Yi
Gu Guan
Hou Jian
Hou Tou
Ma Ji
Mu Guan
Pi Er
Pi San
Pi Yi
Pian Jian
Pian Tou
Qi Li
Qian Tou
San Cha Er
San Cha San
San Cha Yi
Shi Shui
Shui Fu

Shui Zhong
Xiao Jie
Ye Mang
Zeng Chang Er
Zhi Han

Resources

Brad Whisnant can be reached at:

masteringtungacupuncture@yahoo.com
www.sthelensacupuncturist.com
www.masteringtungacupuncture.com

Please sign up for our mailing list to be notified of new books and training sessions.

THE CRANE HERB COMPANIES

Crane Herb Company, Inc.
745 Falmouth Road
Mashpee, MA 02649
Tel: 508-539-1700

info@craneherb.com
www.craneherb.com

Crane-West Herb Pharmacy, Inc.
515 South Main St.
Sebastopol, CA 95472
Tel: 707-823-5691

crane-west@craneherb.com

Crane Herbs provides over 38 brands of Chinese herbs, as of this writing. They also offer ten brands of acupuncture needles. They carry many types of acupuncture supplies. They offer drop shipping direct to your patient or family member via their patient pharmacy. They also offer a custom pharmacy.

Please note that Crane Herb Company *only* sells to state-licensed, and nationally certified Chinese medicine practitioners. **They do not sell to the public.**

REFERENCES

Practical Atlas of Tung's Acupuncture – 2014
Henry McCann and Hans-Georg Ross

Acupuncture 1, 2, 3
Dr. Tan's Strategy of 12 Magical Points
Twelve & Twelve in Acupuncture
Twenty-Four More in Acupuncture
Richard Teh-Fu Tan and Stephen Rush, OMD, LAc.

Lectures on Tung's Acupuncture – Points Study, 2008
Tung's Acupuncture, 2005
Lectures on Tung's Acupuncture Therapeutic System, 2008
Dr. Wei Chieh Young

Introduction to Tung's Acupuncture – 2014
Dr. Chuan-Min Wang DC L.Ac. (Author), Steven Vasilakis LAc (Editor)

Advanced Tung Style Acupuncture: The Dao Ma Needling Technique of Master Tung Ching Chang
James H. Maher

Master Tung's Acupuncture: An Ancient Alternative Style in Modern Clinical Practice, Oct 1992
Miriam Lee

Jing Jin: Acupuncture Treatment of the Muscular System using the Meridian Sinews Paperback – 2010
David Legge

REFERENCES

The Yellow Emperor's Classic of Medicine: A New Translation of the Neijing Suwen with Commentary Paperback – May 10, 1995
Maoshing Ni

Dao of Chinese Medicine: Understanding an Ancient Healing Art Hardcover – August 15, 2002
Donald Edward Kendall

Mapping the Mind Paperback – August 18, 2010
Rita Carter

A Manual of Neuro-Anatomical Acupuncture, Volume I: Musculo-Skeletal Disorders Paperback – January 1, 1999
Joseph Y. Wong

Fundamentals of Chinese Acupuncture (Paradigm title) Paperback – February 1991
Andrew Ellis, Nigel Wiseman, Ken Boss

Twenty-Four More in Acupuncture: Unique Point Applications and Case Studies for Effective Pain Treatment Paperback – 1994
Richard Teh-Fu Tan, Stephen C. Rush

Chapter seven

IMAGES

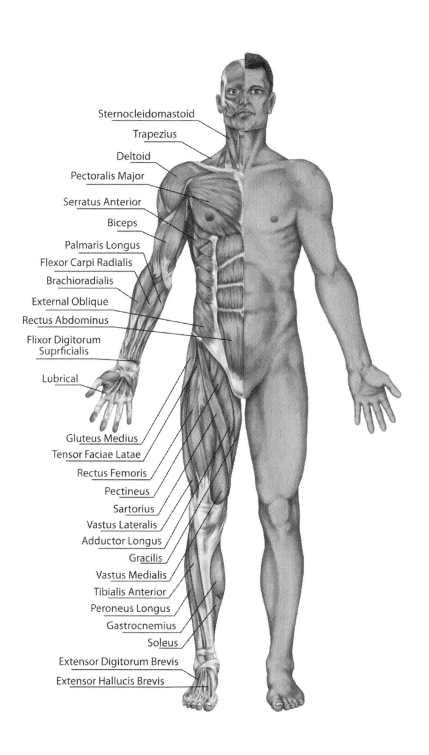

Sternocleidomastoid
Trapezius
Deltoid
Pectoralis Major
Serratus Anterior
Biceps
Palmaris Longus
Flexor Carpi Radialis
Brachioradialis
External Oblique
Rectus Abdominus
Flixor Digitorum Suprficialis
Lubrical
Gluteus Medius
Tensor Faciae Latae
Rectus Femoris
Pectineus
Sartorius
Vastus Lateralis
Adductor Longus
Gracilis
Vastus Medialis
Tibialis Anterior
Peroneus Longus
Gastrocnemius
Soleus
Extensor Digitorum Brevis
Extensor Hallucis Brevis

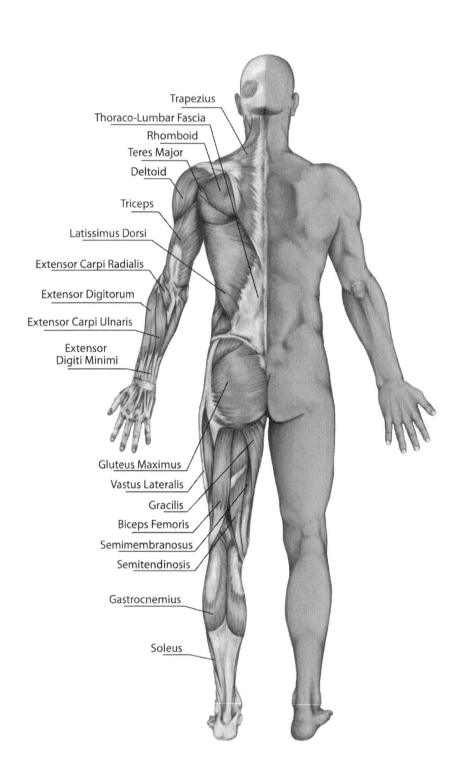

Trapezius

Thoraco-Lumbar Fascia

Rhomboid

Teres Major

Deltoid

Triceps

Latissimus Dorsi

Extensor Carpi Radialis

Extensor Digitorum

Extensor Carpi Ulnaris

Extensor
Digiti Minimi

Gluteus Maximus

Vastus Lateralis

Gracilis

Biceps Femoris

Semimembranosus

Semitendinosis

Gastrocnemius

Soleus

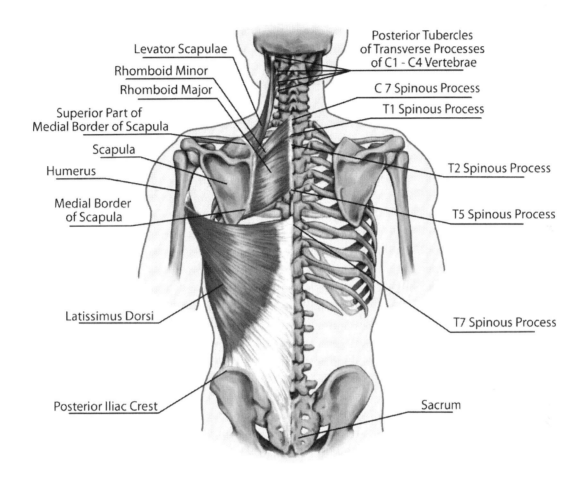

Levator Scapulae

Rhomboid Minor

Rhomboid Major

Superior Part of
Medial Border of Scapula

Scapula

Humerus

Medial Border
of Scapula

Latissimus Dorsi

Posterior Iliac Crest

Posterior Tubercles
of Transverse Processes
of C1 - C4 Vertebrae

C 7 Spinous Process

T1 Spinous Process

T2 Spinous Process

T5 Spinous Process

T7 Spinous Process

Sacrum

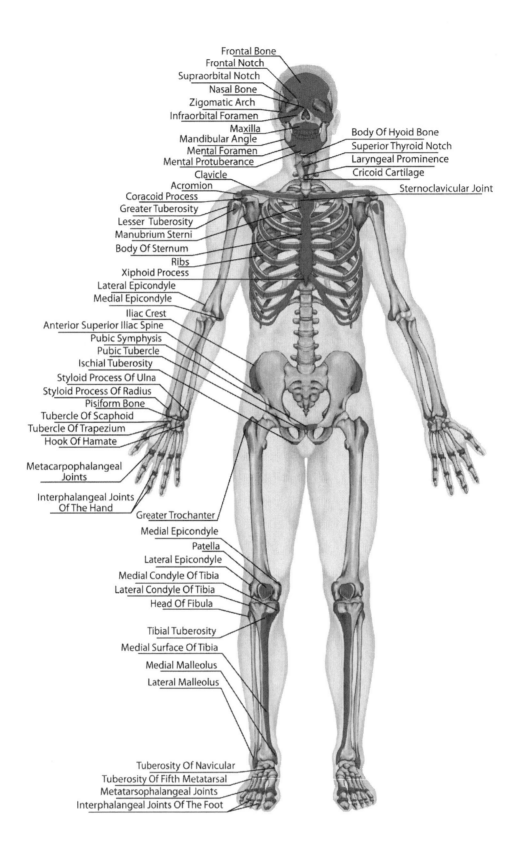

Frontal Bone
Frontal Notch
Supraorbital Notch
Nasal Bone
Zigomatic Arch
Infraorbital Foramen
Maxilla
Mandibular Angle
Mental Foramen
Mental Protuberance
Clavicle
Acromion
Coracoid Process
Greater Tuberosity
Lesser Tuberosity
Manubrium Sterni
Body Of Sternum
Ribs
Xiphoid Process
Lateral Epicondyle
Medial Epicondyle
Iliac Crest
Anterior Superior Iliac Spine
Pubic Symphysis
Pubic Tubercle
Ischial Tuberosity
Styloid Process Of Ulna
Styloid Process Of Radius
Pisiform Bone
Tubercle Of Scaphoid
Tubercle Of Trapezium
Hook Of Hamate
Metacarpophalangeal Joints
Interphalangeal Joints Of The Hand
Greater Trochanter
Medial Epicondyle
Patella
Lateral Epicondyle
Medial Condyle Of Tibia
Lateral Condyle Of Tibia
Head Of Fibula
Tibial Tuberosity
Medial Surface Of Tibia
Medial Malleolus
Lateral Malleolus
Tuberosity Of Navicular
Tuberosity Of Fifth Metatarsal
Metatarsophalangeal Joints
Interphalangeal Joints Of The Foot

Body Of Hyoid Bone
Superior Thyroid Notch
Laryngeal Prominence
Cricoid Cartilage
Sternoclavicular Joint

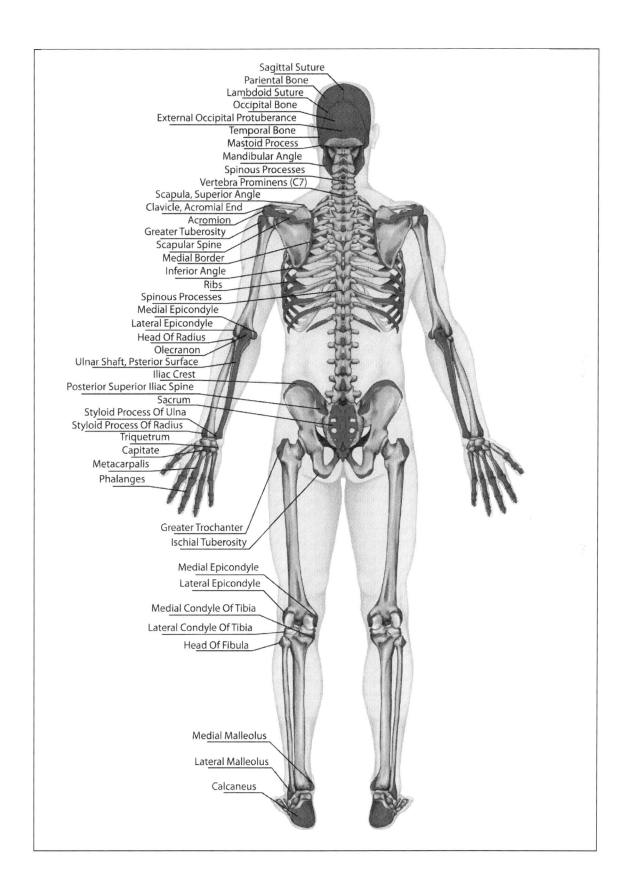

Sagittal Suture
Pariental Bone
Lambdoid Suture
Occipital Bone
External Occipital Protuberance
Temporal Bone
Mastoid Process
Mandibular Angle
Spinous Processes
Vertebra Prominens (C7)
Scapula, Superior Angle
Clavicle, Acromial End
Acromion
Greater Tuberosity
Scapular Spine
Medial Border
Inferior Angle
Ribs
Spinous Processes
Medial Epicondyle
Lateral Epicondyle
Head Of Radius
Olecranon
Ulnar Shaft, Psterior Surface
Iliac Crest
Posterior Superior Iliac Spine
Sacrum
Styloid Process Of Ulna
Styloid Process Of Radius
Triquetrum
Capitate
Metacarpalis
Phalanges

Greater Trochanter
Ischial Tuberosity

Medial Epicondyle
Lateral Epicondyle
Medial Condyle Of Tibia
Lateral Condyle Of Tibia
Head Of Fibula

Medial Malleolus
Lateral Malleolus
Calcaneus

161

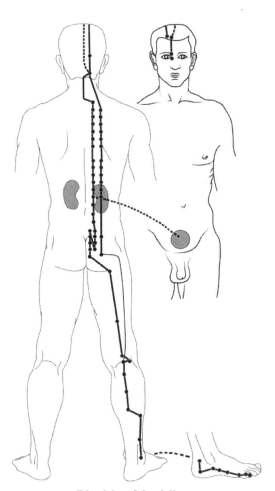

Bladder Meridian

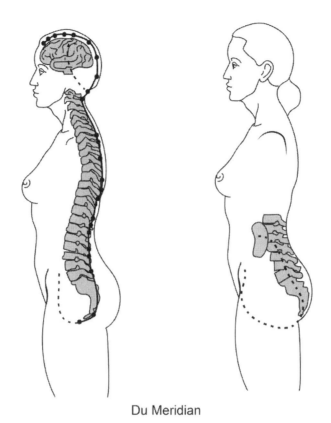

Du Meridian

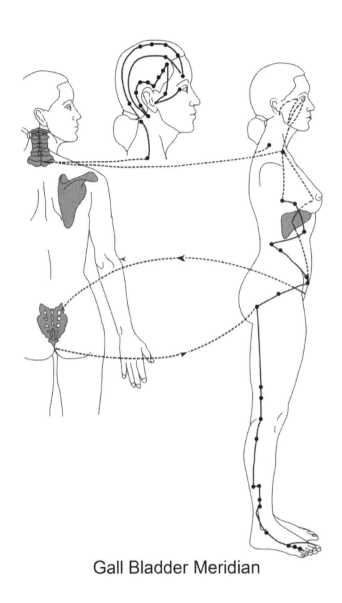

Gall Bladder Meridian

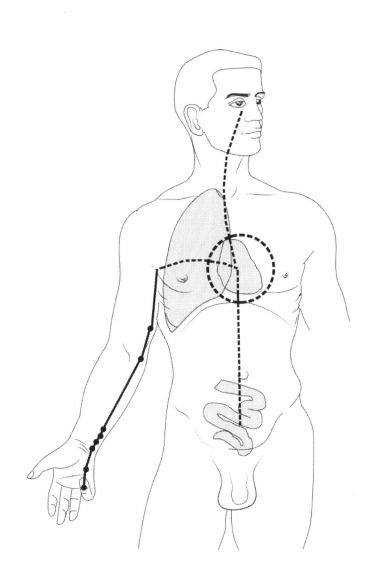

Heart Meridian

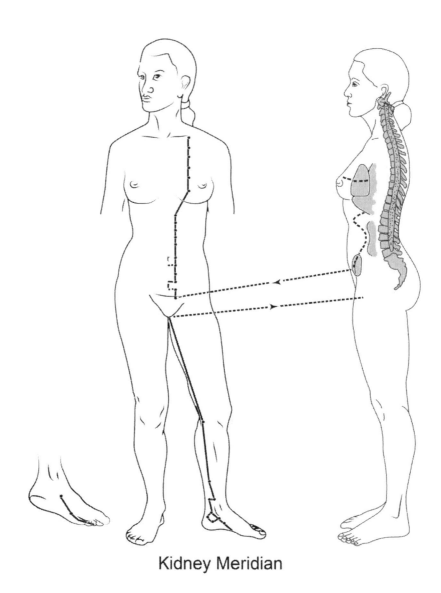

Kidney Meridian

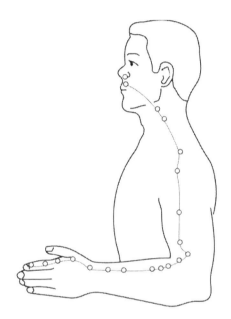 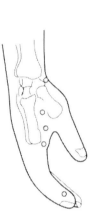

Large Intestine Meridian

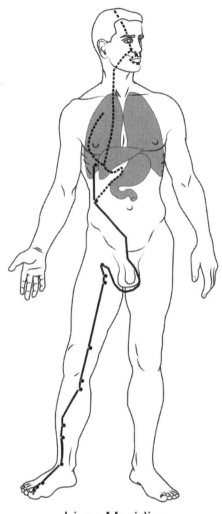

Liver Meridian

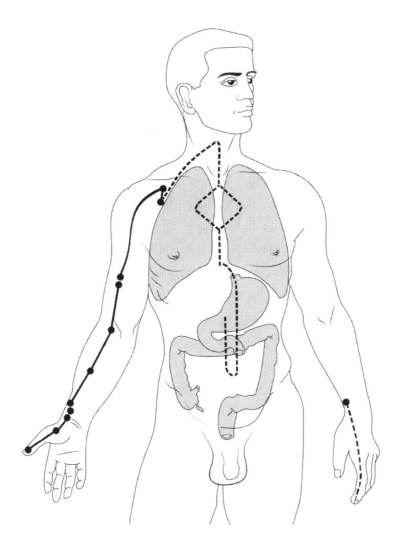

Lung Meridian

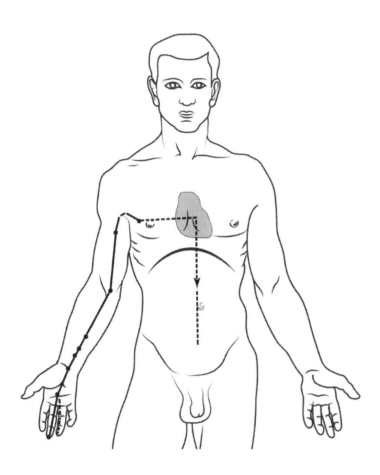

Pericardium Meridian

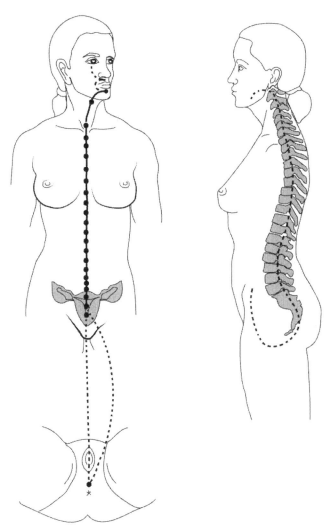

Conception Vessel

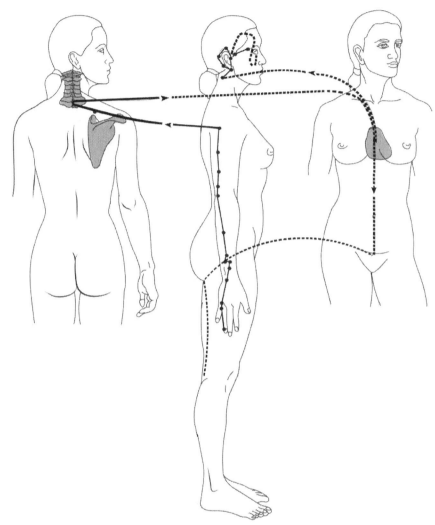

San Jiao Meridian

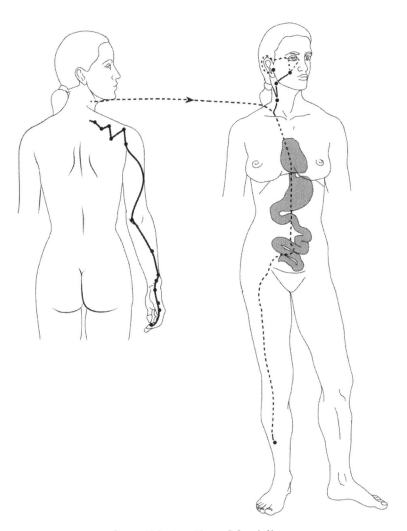

Small Intestine Meridian

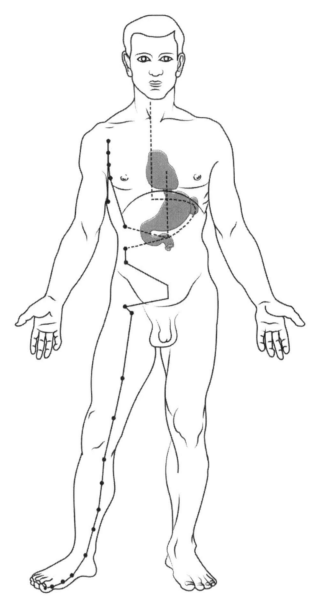

Spleen Meridian

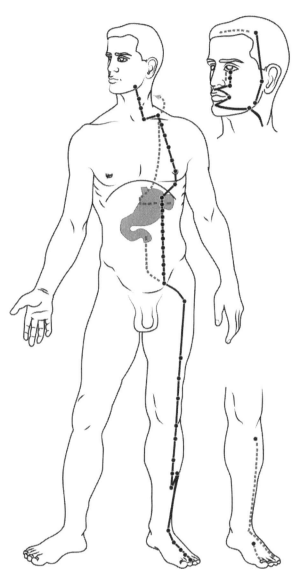

Stomach Meridian

It gives me great pleasure indeed to see the stubbornness of an incorrigible nonconformist warmly acclaimed.

Albert Einstein

Index

Printed in Great Britain
by Amazon